THE RUNNER'S DIET

Recommended Reading:
Runner's World Magazine, $9.50/year
Write for a free catalog of publications
and supplies for runners and other athletes.

Contents

Foreword
Joe Henderson

We hear all kinds of stories and end up wondering what to believe. At one extreme, runners say they couldn't keep training and racing without their organic, unadulterated diets. At the other, Olympic marathoners report living on pizza and beer, and running on defizzed Coke.

Diets of equally successful runners vary so widely—from vegetarian to vitamin J (for junk food)—that the normal conclusion one might draw is, "It doesn't really make any difference what I eat."

If we judge diets by the running results they give, "acceptable" eating habits obviously aren't limited to a few bland items. We can work well with many different fuels, even though some are more effective than others. Because so many factors—chiefly, physical and mental training—contribute to performance, the quantitative differences between different types of food are hard to measure.

However, certain specific dietary adjustments are known to have direct, measurable effects on running. Some involve adding things; more require taking things away.

The most important addition is liquids—particularly for long-distance runners. In events lasting more than an hour, drinks not only enhance performance but protect health itself. Marathon-type runners drink immediately before and during races and long training runs. They can get by on plain water, but water-sugar-salt mixtures put back more of what runners lose.

Carbohydrate-loading—the popular practice of stoking up on bread, spaghetti, and the like before competition—adds extra fuel *before* a runner loses it. Its greatest benefit is in the marathon, where researchers claim it can make five to ten minutes difference in a three-hour runner's time. But its effects diminished with decreased distance, until it has little influence in races of less than ten miles.

Many times, what runners *don't* eat is more important than what they do. Below are a few examples:

Timing. The prerace meal is more ritual than nutritional. It contributes little to the energy output of the event, and the potential for trouble is high when one puts food into a nervous stomach. Many runners prefer to leave well enough alone, staying a little hungry instead of getting a little ill.

Intolerances. Food allergies are common—so common that we may not even recognize them until we combine a hard-to-handle item with a hard run. Some people can't take chocolate or coffee, others apples. Surprisingly common are intolerances to milk and bread. Runners must learn what they are allergic to, and avoid such foods at critical times.

Weight. The big problem in nutrition is not deficiency but overabundance—in this case too much eating, leading to excess weight. Every pound above ideal (and the "ideal" for runners is much less than the one shown on doctors' charts) is an extra burden to carry. It causes a drag on mechanical and oxygen-processing efficiency. The easiest way to improve one's running is to lose a few pounds.

This booklet (originally published in 1972 and one of the most popular in World Publications' library) centers on dietary additions and subtractions that offer runners noticeable benefits.

Certain things do offer hope of improvement. But be careful not to rely on diet too heavily. Food and drink are beginnings, not ends. They aren't substitutes for work or shortcuts to success, but are catalysts that promote the work that opens the way to success.

Joe Henderson

(Joe Henderson wrote all chapters in this book not attributed specifically to other authors.)

Part I
Ingredients of Fitness

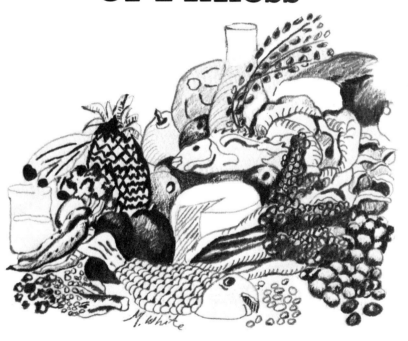

1
To Eat or Not to Eat
Ian Jackson

At age 37, Meinrad Nagele was overweight and out of shape. At age 46, he ran a 2:29 marathon, finishing fourth in the World Veterans championship. After that race, Meinrad wrote, "The vast improvement I attribute to endurance training carried out consistently over a period of many years, together with a special diet (involving natural foods and fasting). This combination is the only method guaranteed to permit acquisition of the highest possible endurance potential."

I knew from personal experience that endurance training worked. So when I read Meinrad's statement that a *combination* of endurance training and a special diet was required, I thought it would be well worth my while to look into the dietary angle.

I knew nothing about "natural foods and fasting." I had assumed that all foods were natural, and I connected fasting with Biblical characters and mystics. It seemed to me that a runner, with his high daily energy expenditure, needed to eat more rather than to abstain from food. After reading around, however, I learned that the kind of "special diet" Meinrad recommended was used by several first-class athletes.

From *Faith, Love and Seaweed* by Ian Rose, I learned about the diet of Murray Rose—the author's son—who was a triple gold-medal winner in the 1956 Olympics, and who repeated with a gold medal for 400 meters in 1960. Murray was a complete vegetarian, never having tasted meat, and he used occasional days of juice fasting as part of his training. From the same book, I learned that Herb Elliott—probably through the influence of Percy Cerutty—was also on a natural foods diet. I remembered that Amby Burfoot, winner of the 1968 Boston marathon, was a vegetarian. I read in the July 1970

edition of *Condition* that six of the top 10 finishers at the
World Veterans marathon were vegetarians. I read in
Runner's World that Erik Ostbye, a Swedish senior marathoner who has run close to 2:20, used fasting during the
last few days before a big race. And, of course, I read the
recommendations of Dr. van Aaken.

I agree that each runner is an "experiment of one" who,
rather than blindly following the training schedules of cham-
pions, should constantly be testing and refining ways of reaching his own performance potential. After gaining confidence
in natural foods and fasting through reading, I decided to
expand my own experiment of one into the dietary field.

EXPERIMENTS IN FASTING

I tried fasting first, because it had the appeal of un-
familiarity. I had a light dinner one evening, consumed
nothing but water throughout the next day, and broke the fast
following my morning run on the third day. In this fast,
and in all subsequent fasts, I continued with the same training
mileage I had been maintaining. But I was careful to run as
efficiently as possible, to conserve energy. I went on a 36-hour
fast once a week for four consecutive weeks. The last one was
on the day before a marathon-distance run, as recommended
by Dr. van Aaken.

For the most part, I felt better when fasting than I usually
do when eating. I felt more alert, lighter on my feet, and more
calm and collected than usual. The only unpleasantness was in
occasional brief periods of weakness and barely noticeable
headaches. These are said to be a sign that the fast is working—that the body is consuming its own nonessential tissues
and, in the process, is flushing out toxic residues into the
bloodstream. (For instance, when fatty tissues are consumed,
the accumulated DDT residues reenter the bloodstream, and
you feel the symptoms of DDT poisoning until the blood has
passed through the kidneys and the DDT has been filtered
into the bladder for excretion.) Luckily, these unpleasant
periods are usually short, lasting only 15-30 minutes. The best
thing is to lie down and rest until they pass. Authorities on
fasting point out that healthy people have a far easier time
than the sick or overweight, and my own experiences support
these observations.

On the whole, I have found going without food to be a fascinating experience. It was amusing to compare the reactions of people I knew. Those who were aware that I was fasting would always greet me with worried comments about how haggard and sickly I looked. Others made surprised remarks about how suddenly I had become "racing fit" and how lean and strong I looked.

After the cautious experimentation with the first 36-hour fast, I decided to try a longer one. I had originally intended to go for 48 or 60 hours. But I felt so much better day after day that I kept extending the limit. Finally, after seven full days, I broke the fast. I wasn't having any difficulties, and as a matter of fact, I was really enjoying myself. I simply thought it would be wiser to wait until I had more experience before going on a longer fast.

Those seven days were such a remarkable experience that it is worth citing some comments from my running log. (I keep the log by elapsed time—in parentheses—rather than distance. The pace on these runs ranged from under 6:00 per mile to about 7:30.)

March 15 (2:30) "... pulse 33 at rest (evening)."
March 16 (2:10) "... felt vaguely (very vaguely) headachy."
March 17 (2:30) "... felt much stronger today than I did yesterday."
March 18 (1:55) (I ran in a 20-mile March of Dimes walkathon with Rich Delgado. We went off course for an additional mile or so.) "I was amazed to hear Rich say that he thought we were well under a 2:30 marathon pace and that his legs were sore. I have fasted since Tuesday and yet the pace felt easy. I feel I could have picked up the pace over another six miles if I had been in a race."
March 19 (2:35) "... felt all right during the run, but tired and sluggish afterwards."
March 20 (2:00) "... felt mildy fatigued today."
March 21 (2:25) "... fast run. Felt apprehensive about energy level, but I had no problems and I felt strong."

The last day's run was quite an experience. Although the pace got hot, it was absurdly easy to stay with it. I remember experiencing a sense of calm detachment. My body was moving effortlessly, gliding along with no urging. Everything was smooth, mellow, and peaceful. My senses were incredibly heightened, finely tuned in. I felt a natural unity with the dark trees and the drifting mist. The sighing of the wind in the pines, the clear bird calls, and the occasional creaking of branches seemed to penetrate gently into the very center of my being. With a combination of elation and gratitude, I let my body move on while my mind and my senses touched their home.

When we began the long climb out of the park, I had a momentary flash of apprehension. This was the acid test. Surely I wouldn't be able to handle the hills after seven days without food. But the hills presented no difficulties. My body was still gliding, still moving smoothly without any conscious urging. I seemed to be floating up the hills like a feather being wafted by gentled breezes.

Since then, I have had similar experiences on other fasts. As far as I'm concerned, they are reason enough to continue regular, moderate fasting. I don't know what they should be called. A psychologist would probably come up with something like "psycho-spiritual enhancement." I would call them pure awareness of joyful existence.

But I think that competitive performances could also be improved through fasting. I have often wondered what would have happened if I had been running a marathon on that seventh day of fasting. I have a feeling I would have been capable of a very good time since I seemed to have unlimited speed and endurance. But I am not an expert on fasting, nor, for that matter, on the natural foods diet. Anyone who is interested can soon learn as much as I know simply by reading the books listing at the end of this article and by trying some of these things himself.

HOW FASTING WORKS

I'm sure there is a lot of controversy about the theoretical grounds of fasting and natural foods, just as there is about training theories. But why should we runners wait for a resolution of theoretical matters? We don't need to. A little personal experimentation is worth far more than volumes of theoretical discussions.

I asked Meinrad Nagele about a controversial aspect of vegetarian diet. He gave me a wry smile and said, "Who knows? Diet is a battlefield." He's absolutely right. Nutrition is such a young science and so full of uncertainties that we'll get nowhere if we wait for absolute scientific validation of dietary practices. But what's to stop us from trying a few unconventional approaches? Certainly no harm can come from eating natural foods. And—provided you inform yourself about fasting and try it cautiously—no harm can come from it, either. My own experiences aren't unusual; anyone making the same dietary experiments will find out that running is easier this way.

I haven't been able to find an explanation of why running becomes easier with fasting. But I can think of two possible answers.

1. The first is obvious. When you lose weight, your power-to-weight ratio improves, and you can maintain a faster average pace. Not only do you save the work of carrying unnecessary tissues. You also conserve the oxygen that would otherwise have been used to supply them. For these reasons, Dr. van Aaken has been recommending weight loss for many years.

2. The second answer is not so obvious. It involves the reduction of internal "friction." I am not qualified to judge its scientific validity, but it sounds plausible.

Running efficiency is based ultimately on metabolic efficiency, which involves the processing of raw materials (air, water, food) to produce energy. As by-products of the metabolic processes, many waste materials are formed. If everything is in order, the waste materials are eliminated through sweat, urine, feces, and exhaled air. But if metabolism is inefficient, residual wastes can accumulate in the cells and tissues, and create obstructions by their presence. For instance, uric acid—a waste product caused by excessive protein consumption—can form a crystalline structure that lodges in the tissues. Some other undesirable accumulations are carbonic acid, cholesterol, chlorine, and calcium carbonate. Most of these waste products are found in the connective tissues. But they can also end up in organs, glands, and nerve coverings. German physicians have termed these products *Zellen-schlacken*, or "cell cinders."

Now consider the bloodstream, the medium through which the metabolic process is carried out. It transports nutritive elements and oxygen to the cells, and carries waste products—including carbon dioxide—to the organs of elimination (the lungs, the bowels, the kidneys, and the skin). Blood does not actually enter into the cells, but makes the exchange through osmosis—permeation through the porous cell membranes. If the cell membranes are partially blocked by waste products, such as cholesterol, osmosis, and consequently metabolism, become inefficient. Inefficient metabolism affects all body functions, including running.

During a fast, the body must consume its own tissues to provide energy. This is known as *autolysis*. The body is amazingly precise in the selection of tissues, consuming them in the reverse order of importance. Fat tissues, tumors, and accumulated residual wastes are first to go. What cannot be used for energy is flushed out of the body, primarily through the urine. The more internal obstructions are flushed out, the greater the reduction of internal "friction," and the greater the improvement in metabolic efficiency. With improved metabolic efficiency, a runner is capable of coming closer to his performance potential.

Once the internal cleansing has been started through regular, moderate fasting, it should be helped along by the avoidance of dietary habits that tend to produce more residual wastes. This is where natural foods come in.

WAERLAND NATURAL FOODS DIET

Natural foods are simply foods that have not been tampered with in any way—that have not been refined or processed, that have not been adulterated by the addition of artificial flavors and colors, or chemical preservatives. The natural foods diet involves fresh fruits and vegetables, whole grains, nuts and seeds, raw milk products, and raw honey.

I made many mistakes when I began the transition to natural foods. Fresh fruit sounded appetizing, and so did raw honey and things made with it. But vegetables didn't appeal to me at all. I started living on fruit, honey ice cream, carob bars, halvah, and honeycomb. I ate haphazardly, and I ate too much. Pretty soon I realized that I didn't feel any better than before, except when I was fasting. When I was eating, I felt bloated and sluggish. I was about to give up the natural foods idea when I had the good fortune to meet Meinrad Nagele, whose comment about a special diet had originally sparked my interest.

We talked extensively on training and diet, and I came to recognize my mistakes. His special diet is the *Waerland diet,* which is famous in Europe but almost unknown in the United States. He told me that Erik Ostbye was on the diet, too. I learned that it is not enough to eat a few good foods. You must be sure that there is enough variety to provide balanced nutrition. The Waerland diet has proved its effectiveness with thousands of Europeans over the past few decades. There is no need to worry about missing some nutritive element if you follow its pattern carefully.

The diet was developed over 20 years ago by Are Waerland, an unusually energetic, brilliant scholar of Swedish descent. The diet itself is only part of a biologically correct system of living, which includes plenty of fresh air, sunshine, and aerobic exercise. It involves avoiding all table salt and cooking salt (there is plenty of the right kind of salt in vegetables), as well as coffee, strong tea, drinking at meals, very hot drinks, tobacco, alcohol, sweets, chocolate, white bread and cakes made of white flour, meat, fish, and eggs.

Incidentally, the Waerland diet is surprisingly inexpensive. It costs far less than a conventional diet. Whole grains, for instance, cost only 8-12 cents a pound. Any whole food is usually cheaper than a refined, processed, and packaged food. The reason is obvious. The more the food is handled, the more it will cost because the processors must make a profit. Ironically, the expensive, processed foods are also inferior nutritionally. You end up paying more for less food value.

Breakfast. Since the body is eliminating waste products up to about noon, the breakfast is a light, easily digested meal of fresh fruit and sour milk. This goes against the current emphasis on eating heavy, high-protein breakfasts, but my own experience suggests that a light breakfast is wiser. I usually run before breakfast, sometimes in the 20- to 30-mile range. And yet a light fruit breakfast gives me far more energy than the high-protein breakfasts I used to eat.

Lunch. This is a whole-grain cereal called Kruska. The whole grains (wheat, barley, rye, oats, and millet) are ground up immediately before cooking in order to preserve the nutritive elements. Exposure to air destroys enzymes and plant hormones.

Dinner. The Waerland dinner is based on potatoes, baked or boiled in their skins, or mashed, with raw beets and carrots grated over them. In addition, there is a large helping of salad greens and sour milk. Everything except for the cereals and the potatoes is eaten raw, because all processing—including cooking—reduces nutritive value.

When I first saw what the diet involved, I groaned inwardly. Except for the fruit breakfast, it seemed bland and unappetizing. Now, I'm surprised how much I look forward to each meal. Perhaps my taste buds have been somehow sensitized by cutting out all foods with chemical additives. For the first time in my life, I find that I really relish vegetables.

The diet is so simple, appetizing, inexpensive, and health-inducing that I think it worthy of the attention of all runners. If Hans Selye is right about the effects of stress, anything that reduces stress will enable a runner to train and race with less chance of breakdown. The Waerland diet reduces the stress of internal waste products. I have no idea of the racing improvement to be expected. But I'm sure that increased biologic strength must make a difference, if only indirectly, by improving stress tolerance so that a heavier training load can be handled without fear of stress injuries.

I encourage you to give it a try. Only by experimentation will we be able to find out if diet is a factor in running performance. If the ideas I have presented here are worthless, let's prove them so by exposing their ineffectiveness. But don't condemn them before you've looked into them. If you venture to expand your experiment of one to include diet, you can only gain. No matter what results you get, you'll be more aware of your own needs and your approach to running will be more comprehensive, more intelligent.

We runners have all had plenty of the petty persecution from the unenlightened. We have all endured snears and cat-calls during our training runs. Surely we can put up with a little ridicule about "food fanaticism," too. You already know that the cat-callers have no idea what they're missing in running. I think you'll find the same thing when you try natural foods and fasting.

References

Airola, Paavo. *Health Secrets from Europe.* New York: Arc Books, 1971.
Rose, Ian. *Faith, Love and Seaweed.* New York: Award Books.
Shelton, Herbert. *Fasting Can Save Your Life.* Chicago: Natural Hygiene Press, 1964.
Shelton, Herbert. *Food Combining Made Easy.* Chicago: Natural Hygiene Press, 1951.
Waerland, Ebba. *Rebuilding Health.* New York: Arc Books, 1968.

2
Dietary Essentials

The best way to start talking about sound athletic nutrition is to first talk about sound *human* nutrition. The athlete's basic needs aren't significantly different than those of other healthy persons. We're all bound by the same broad dietary laws.

This chapter spells out some of those laws, a necessary framework for understanding the specifics of running diet that come later. This isn't meant to be a complete course in nutrition, only an introduction in simplest terms. Some factors are skipped over lightly, or are ignored altogether—either because they're too obvious to mention, or have little direct bearing on the runner.

In this introduction, indeed throughout the book, keep several points in mind.

1. Athletes live within the same general dietary boundaries as all other people. The "goods" and the "bads" are basically the same for all groups, although there are some subtle differences in food tastes and tolerances.

2. "Normal" nutrition covers a broad range of eating and drinking possibilities. There are literally millions of combinations of nutrients that satisfy human wants and needs.

3. Eating is one of the joys of life. Since there are so many routes to the same end—good nutrition—we're free within the limits of food availability to choose things that are good to eat, not just *good for us*. With creative eating, the kind of dietary control often recommended for runners need not be a chore.

4. The human body is an amazingly sensitive instrument. Through clear physical symptoms, it makes known what it thrives on and what it doesn't want. It takes and uses what

it needs and rejects the rest. The runner, attempting to operate at peak efficiency, is uniquely tuned in to the body's reactions to food and drink. Sometimes the effect is pleasant, sometimes not, and this is usually more noticeable to runners than to people operating at less than their best.

FOODS AND FUNCTIONS

Everything we take in by mouth and send on the long, complicated trip through the digestive system serves one or more of the following purposes: (1) *growth*—building and/or repairing tissues; (2) *energy production*—providing heat and power for work; (3) *control*—regulating body processes.

Six classes of nutrients do these jobs:

1. Carbohydrates: Starchy, sugary compounds that act as energy sources.
2. Fats: Oily substances that also provide energy.
3. Proteins: Found in most concentrated form in meats, proteins are primarily growth promoters but also aid energy-production and body control.
4. Minerals: Promote growth and control. Some of the most important minerals to the runner are iron, magnesium, potassium, calcium, and sodium.
5. Vitamins: Crucial forces in the body's regulation and growth systems. Key vitamins for runners are A, C, E, and the B-complex group (thiamin, riboflavin, niacin, etc.).
6. Water: Growth and control factor.

Water, carbohydrates, fats, and proteins are by far the most abundant substances in food. Most foods are combinations of these four. Minerals and vitamins are present in only tiny amounts—so small, in fact, that some of them have just recently been identified. Humans need all of these nutrients in certain minimum quantities to sustain healthy life.

CALORIES AND WEIGHT

Total food intake is measured in calories. Scientifically speaking, a *calorie* is "the amount of heat required to raise the temperature of one kilogram of water one degree centigrade." Nutritionally speaking, calories are the currency one must take in and save to gain weight, or to avoid and spend to lose it. One pound of body weight contains about 3,500 calories of energy. To gain a pound, one must take in and store that many calories. To lose a pound, the reverse is true: get rid of what is stored.

All activities burn up calories. Even sitting in a rocking chair reading the newspaper uses them at the rate of about a quarter-calorie per pound per hour. Moderate exercise, such as working in the garden, uses about a half-calorie per pound per hour. "Severe" exercise, according to one physiology textbook, consumes one full calorie per pound per hour—or more. Running is even more "severe" than this textbook indicates. Researchers have found that a long-distance runner uses calories at the rate of perhaps 1,000 an hour (more than 5 per pound). Sprinters burn 10 times that much, but only for brief periods. But still, on running alone, it takes as much as 35 miles of running to lose a single pound.

All carbohydrate, fat, and protein foods contain calories; water, minerals, and vitamins do not. For moderately active mature adults, the recommended caloric intake is about 18 per pound per day for men, and about 16 for women. This totals about 2,700 per day for a 150-pound man, and 2,000 a day for a 125-pound woman. Obviously, though, daily calorie intake can't be reduced to a formula that applies to everyone. Each individual has to make himself what Dr. George Sheehan calls "an experiment of one." Determine your own needs.

Weight is the best guide. Decide the weight at which you run best; then try to get up or down to it, and maintain it. It's as simple as balancing caloric intake with energy expenditure. It's simple *on paper,* that is. In practice, this isn't so easy. Low weight is unquestionably an advantage in running. Eating isn't like filling a grocery bag. The excess food we put in ourselves doesn't fall out on the ground. It stays in storage to be carried along as an extra load. The general populace eats and weighs too much. Surprisingly, within the context of their exercise many runners also eat and weigh too much.

Dr. Irwin Stillman, author of *The Doctor's Quick Weight Loss Diet,* has devised the best formula yet for figuring weight.

Runners can use it to check themselves. The Stillman formula is this:

> Men use 110 pounds and five feet as a base; for each inch over five feet, add 5½ pounds. This gives an "average" weight for a man's height. Stillman says the "ideal" figure would be about 10 percent less. For instance, an average 6'0" man would weigh 170 pounds; his ideal weight would be 151-52. For women, the base figures are 100 pounds and five feet; and five pounds for each each additional inch. The rest of the calculations are the same.

Runners in the sprints tend to be somewhere between the "average" and "ideal" levels, and middle- and long-distance athletes usually are even lighter than the ideal. If weight is above average, some caloric balancing apparently needs to be done. (More on this in a later chapter.)

Proper eating, however, is more subtle than simply shoveling in the food at hand until you can hold no more. There are a number of other factors to consider. Total food intake is one among many.

RECOMMENDED DAILY ALLOWANCES

Nutrition is a relatively new science, still in a shifting state. This much is evident from looking at the U.S. national dietary recommendations. Before 1943 there weren't any recognized ones. Then that year the Food and Nutrition Board of the National Academy of Sciences began publishing its Recommended Daily Allowances (RDAs) for calories, proteins, vitamins, and minerals. The present recommendations are very different from the original ones. That's because the RDAs have been reviewed constantly since 1943, with revisions to the list published every five years. In theory, each revision is an improvement.

The 1974 figures are the latest ones released by the Food and Nutrition Board. (See chart in the Appendix.) The recommendations are not minimums, maximums, or absolutes. They are merely guidelines or averages, which if followed provide adequate nutrition—and then some. According to the board, they "afford a margin sufficiently above average physiological requirements to cover variations among practically all individuals in the general population. The allowances provide a buffer against increased needs during common stresses and permit full realization of growth and productive potential. But they are not necessarily adequate to meet the additional requirements of persons depleted by disease, traumatic stress or prior dietary inadequacies."

In other words, these are educated guesses based on an elusive "average, healthy" person. What about the runner, who is somewhat abnormal in his activity and may at the same time be both unhealthy and super-healthy? The answer here isn't so clear, and is the source of much of the controversy surrounding athletes' diets. The question of whether or not athletes need special diets because of their special stresses hasn't been fully explored scientifically, and so as yet is far from fully answered. We will explore some clues later in this book. The chart on the following page offers some conventional recommendations. Runners shouldn't stray far from them.

ESSENTIAL NUTRIENTS

To review, the six main elements of the diet are carbohydrates, fats, proteins, minerals, vitamins, and water. They're present, in varying degrees and combinations, in foods and drinks. Here we'll talk briefly about what they do and where they're found.

Carbohydrates. These are the high-energy foods, primarily the sugars and starches. Their energy characteristics give them utmost importance for running. Carbohydrate products are the main fuel in relatively short, fast bursts of energy, because they can be used quickly and efficiently. When carbohydrates break down they wind up as glycogen—a substance stored in limited amounts in the liver and muscles. Glycogen burns vigorously during exercise, but since the supply is limited it may run out before the end of the run. Loading the diet with carbohydrates can increase the glycogen supply to a certain extent. Almost all foods have proportionately more carbohydrates than fats or proteins. Sugars and cereal grains are the most common sources.

Fats. Because of the connection with obesity, fats have

gotten a bad name. In fact, they're the best source of energy that the body has, being more concentrated than carbohydrates. However, during heavy exercise fats break down slower than the carbohydrates. In high stress situations, fats simply aren't as efficient. Animal fats and vegetable oils are the richest sources of this essential nutrient.

Proteins. They are the body-builders, helping bones and tissues grow and repair themselves. The body needs a considerable amount of protein to keep operating smoothly. According to the Food and Nutrition Board, an adult needs 0.9 gram a day per kilogram of body weight (this translates to 0.33 gram per pound). These complex substances are available in a number of forms. The most obvious are fish and meat, which contain high quality, concentrated protein. The best are beef, chicken, pork chops, liver, haddock, and salmon. However, protein needs can be met entirely without eating meats (as a number of vegetarians illustrate later in this book). Eggs, dairy products, nuts, beans and peas, grains, and cereals are good protein sources.

Minerals. To the runner, the most important ones are those that strongly influence muscular action and oxygen consumption. The muscle-related ones are calcium, phosphorus, sodium, potassium, and magnesium. Iron is invaluable in oxygen transport.

1. *Calcium*, working together with phosphorus, promotes normal action of the heart muscle and helps it maintain a rhythmic beat. Dairy products, oranges, and eggs are rich in calcium.

2. *Phosphorus* is transformed into a chemical compound that helps the body release energy. It is found in dairy products, lean meats and fish, eggs, and whole-grain cereals.

3. *Sodium* and *potassium* have the overlapping functions of maintaining the body's fluid balance and transmitting muscle impulses. Most foods contain sodium naturally. Citrus fruits are rich in potassium.

4. *Magnesium* acts as a transmitter of nerve impulses and as a trigger for muscle contractions. Without it, there are

muscle tremors and cramps. Vegetables, cereals grains, and nuts are good sources.

5. *Iron* is important to the red blood cells, which carry oxygen. When iron supplies are short, anemia (with a generalized feeling of weakness) results. Organ meats (such as liver), dried fruits, dark green vegetables, and eggs provide iron.

Vitamins. The ones that interest runners the most are E (which influences heart action and endurance), C (which builds resistance and speeds healing), and the B-complex vitamins (which promote energy metabolism). Others with established daily recommendations are A (important to eyesight, growth, and resistance) and D (valuable to the bone structure).

1. *Vitamin E* is found naturally in vegetable oils like wheat germ oil.

2. *Vitamin C* (also called ascorbic acid) is present in citrus fruits, broccoli, and selected other fruits and vegetables.

3. Of the B-complex vitamins, *thiamin* (a catalyst in the oxidation of glucose) comes in greatest supply from pork chops, ham, peas, beans, liver, rice, and oatmeal; *riboflavin* (involved in both protein and energy metabolism) is found in liver, meats, milk, and whole grains; *niacin* (mental and physical resistance) is in milk, eggs, meats, and nuts.

Yellow and green vegetables provide *vitamin A.*
Fish liver oils and fortified milk give adequate *vitamin D.*

Water. Since the body is mostly water, it needs a considerable fresh supply each day just to maintain its essential balance and to carry on its functions normally. With water, unlike food, there is little danger of taking too much. Excess food is stored in the form of fat. The kidneys simply flush out excess water.

DIET BALANCING

The Recommended Daily Allowances, taken as a group, make such a mass of figures that it almost takes a slide rule to be sure of meeting all the needs. There's a simpler way to do it, however, than counting every gram, milligram, and international unit. The simplified method is the Basic Four chart that children learn in school and promptly forget. If followed carefully, it should fill most of the needs. The Basic Four chart lumps food into groups: (1) milk group; (2) meat group; (3) vegetable-fruit group; and (4) bread-cereals group. The daily recommendations below are based on standard U.S. eating habits.

Milk Group. Two to three glasses of milk for children under 9; children 9-12—three or more glasses; teenagers—four or more glasses; adults—two or more glasses. (Cheese, ice cream, and other milk-based foods can supply part of the milk.)

Meat Group. Two or three three-ounce servings. (Eggs, cheese, beans, peas, lentils, and nuts may be substituted.)

Vegetable-Fruit Group. Four or more half-cup servings; group includes dark-green or deep-yellow vegetables, citrus fruits, potatoes, and other fruits and vegetables.

Bread-Cereals Group. Four or more servings, preferably whole grains.

Fats, sweets, and flavorings may be added within the limits of individual calorie needs and tastes. However, it is preferable to fill all needs from the basic four. These four provide every essential nutrient. If these foods are eaten regularly, in proper amounts and following proper preparation, there is no need for anything more. Manufactured vitamin and mineral supplements offer nothing that isn't available naturally in foods. And natural foods are the most pleasant way to get your nutrition—if not the cheapest and most effective.

RUNNERS' SPECIAL NEEDS

The runner works harder than the average person, and he does his work in fairly violent bursts lasting from a few seconds to a few hours. While working this way, the demands on his muscular, energy, and fluid systems are higher than normal. To meet these demands, runners need diets that strike three delicate balances:

1. Maintaining energy for a higher than normal output, without so much food that excess is stored as fat.
2. Maintaining the muscle bulk and strength needed for the

higher-than-normal muscular work of the event, without
sacrificing instant energy.

3. Maintaining enough liquid to preserve the body's fluid
   balance, and replacing lost liquids with minerals as well
   as water.

Performance *can* be improved—often dramatically—with
dietary control. There are scientific studies and personal experiences to substantiate it. The three main ways are: (1) by
adjusting the ratio between carbohydrate and fatty foods ver-
sus proteins; (2) by drinking mineral-loading liquids immediately before, during, and after hard runs; and (3) by taking
heavy doses of certain vitamins. To elaborate:

1. Recent scientific evidence shows two things: (a) Heavy
   carbohydrate intake (with a corresponding reduction in
   fats and proteins) before competition greatly improves
   distance-running performance; simply stated, that's
   because carbohydrates are most rapidly converted to
   usable energy. (b) Runners apparently need no more
   protein than nonrunners. Some researchers suggest that
   they need *less* than the customary amount. (The Recommended Daily Allowances call for 25 percent less protein
   than previously listed.)

2. Minerals play a key part in warding off muscle fatigue
   and cramping. Recognizing this fact, manufacturers have
   produced a number of electrolyte replacement drinks in
   recent years. They generally contain sodium chloride,
   calcium, and potassium. Recent research has shown that
   sodium chloride (ordinary table salt) may be less important than previously imagined, and that potassium and
   magnesium losses are the most crucial to the runner. At
   any rate, runners report significant improvements in distance times after taking water-electrolyte-sugar drinks
   during races. The drink that best synthesizes the runner's
   sweat seems to produce the best results.

3. The so-called megavitamins approach to athletic diet is
   still subject to a great deal of controversy. This is the habit
   of gobbling vitamin tablets at rates 10 or more times
   above the Recommended Daily Allowances. The value

and wisdom of this practice are still in the speculative stages. But there is a certain amount of test data suggesting that big doses of vitamin E and vitamin C are worthwhile. Vitamin E is said to affect the heart function and endurance. Vitamin C apparently provides protection against illness and injury, and speeds recovery. There is some truth to the claims that added carbohydrates, minerals, and vitamins benefit the runner. There is a danger, though, in taking the attitude that "if X amount is good for me, double X must then be twice as good." That kind of logic doesn't stand up. The task of the exercise physiologist—as well as the exercising runner—is to discover that perfect X.

3
Too Much of Nothing

Otto Brucker, M.D.

Anyone who enters athletics announces indirectly that he does not want to neglect his body. The athlete, in attempting to maximize performance, realizes that any disturbance in the physical system will be a hindrance. The body's complicated metabolic system has to operate at peak efficiency, and a basic condition for this is fulfilling nutritional needs.

However, the growing number of nutritionally caused diseases, and the high percentage of people afflicted, indicates that the basic nutritional needs of the society are not being adequately met. The widespread concept that athletes can prevent these diseases simply by exercising can be dangerous. This is not to say exercise is not important in the maintenance of health. But the athlete should keep in mind that while a man can stay healthy with proper nutrition without sufficient movement, he *cannot* remain healthy on any amount of exercise if essential nutritional elements are lacking. The ravages of poor nutrition cannot be prevented or softened by any kind of athletic activity. Despite the obvious physical benefits of exercise, it is clear that this activity cannot make up for the lack of essential metabolic substances. The reverse is more often the case. The more intense the physical movement, the more necessary is a sufficient supply of vital substances.

Just what constitutes a "sufficient supply of vital substances" is still open to some question. But a new body of nutritional research is currently replacing (or at least modifying) conventional medical thinking on this subject. Since these new findings have long since passed the stage of theory and have practical application behind them, it seems negligent to continue quoting older nutritional theses. But the most important aspects of the "new nutrition" become clear when contrasted with the old theories (which, though outdated, still influence thinking today).

Old nutritional theory assumed that a supply of the three basic nutritional elements—protein, fat, and carbohydrates—along with certain minerals, was sufficient for health. These were supposed to provide 2,000 to 4,000 calories a day. This measurement of the caloric content of the three basic elements is a mark of the "old nutrition." Not even the discovery of vitamins changed anything important in this basic principle. Vitamins were merely added to the existing list of recommendations.

New nutritionists have discovered, however, that the three basic substances, certain minerals, and the classic vitamins are in no way enough to maintain health and performance capacity. Countless other substances are required, which they refer to as "vital substances." These include not only the generally recognized vitamins and minerals, but also minerals present in the tiniest amounts (called "trace elements"), a large group of enzymes, polyunsaturated fatty acids, and aromatic substances. Some of these are necessary for good health; others must be present for life itself to go on.

The common cause of performance lags and nutritionally associated diseases lies in the incorrect concepts of older nutritional theory. This is expressed as an overemphasis on nutritional concentrates (isolated elements in the diet) and an underestimation of total nutritional needs. Injury to health comes mainly from manufactured nutritional products. These are marked by a lack of vital substances essential to health. The more concentrated the substance, the fewer vital elements it contains, and the more harmful it is to health.

In old nutritional theory, the worth of a diet was measured by its caloric content. In the new order of things, nutrition is based on the diet's vitality. The more food is left to nature, the more alive it is; the less natural, the less lifelike. The scale extends from completely lifeless industrial preparations such as white sugar, to conserved and heated nutrients, to foods in their natural state.

Nutritional researcher Kollath set up a scientifically exact order of preference in his book *The Order of Our Nutrition.* In descending order of vitality these foods include: (1) completely natural; (2) fermentatively altered; (3) mechanically altered; (4) heated; (5) conserved; and (6) prepared (artificially concentrated nutrients).

The two main representatives of isolated nutritional concentrates with insufficient vital substances are (1) white sugar,
and (2) refined flours. Their danger is considerably greater
than is generally recognized, and is based on the following
points:

- They are practically void of vital substances.
- They are eaten daily in large amounts by most people.
- Their harmfulness is still unknown to most people.

The growing number of industrially altered fats also contributes to ill-health. These include margarines and oil
products produced by chemical processes. Other manufactured dietary items play smaller roles because of their low
consumption.

Nutrients that contain no vital substances can be called
"dead foods." In this sense, Kollath distinguishes between
food and "nutritional preparations." He says that "nutritional
preparations" cannot be considered food, since they lack certain essential elements necessary to support life and health.
Food is alive because it contains all substances necessary for
life and health.

"Industrial" sugars cause a harmful chain reaction. Not
only do they lack vital substances; they also act as vitamin
thieves because they require vitamins (particularly B-vitamins)
for their digestion. In addition, these sugars interfere with
some enzyme activity.

It is misleading to say that eating isolated sugars increases
energy. In fact, it requires great energy just to assimilate these
products. Eating these sugars drains away vital substances
while adding none; they disturb enzyme functions, and in the
end do not increase strength and energy levels at all. Eating
isolated sugars is also damaging due to their quick assimilation. Pure sugar, especially dextrose (glucose), passes quickly
through the intestinal walls into the bloodstream. In old
nutritional theory this is viewed as advantageous and desirable. In truth, it has a negative effect. The immediate rise in
blood-sugar is followed by a dramatic drop to levels below
normal. (This is called a *hypoglycemia state.*) If the athlete
tries to boost this back up with further sugar intake, he creates
an even greater imbalance in his blood sugar level.

Athletes should keep in mind that proper metabolism can take place *only* when all the necessary vital substances are delivered, in balanced proportions. This is true of consumption of both sugar and nutritional grain products. Kollath was one of those responsible for the discovery of vital nutritional substances. Through experiments in animals, he succeeded in producing diseases by withholding certain of these nutrients.

Czech scientist Bernasek has gone further with Kollath's experiments. Bernasek has shown that a still larger number of unidentified vitamins exist. He fed rats a purely synthetic diet that contained all previously known vital substances necessary for maintaining life and health. Diseases nevertheless occurred. The most remarkable part of these experiments was that pathological changes in organs were found in the first generation only to a limited degree. But they appeared more and more acutely from generation to generation. Beyond the fifth generation, there was no further reproduction. An equally important result of these tests was that all the damage was preventable by feeding whole grains.

These observations have a further striking parallel to human beings now in the third and fourth generation of *not* eating whole-grain products. Their diets resemble those of the experimental animals insofar as carbohydrates consist predominately of pure starch and sugar preparations, fats are made up of margarines and chemically extracted oils, and proteins are denatured by heating processes. Degenerative phenomena in man—especially in the nervous system—have striking similarities to the pathological findings in rats during Bernasek's experiments.

New nutritionists have uncovered a number of other important facts of great practical significance. The two leading ones are:

- Vegetable proteins are just as valuable as animal proteins.
- Heating contributes to the destruction of proteins.

Researchers Kollath and Bernasek also made key discoveries in the protein area. When protein substances were heated to a maximum of 34° C (93° F), the laboratory rats lived normally. But when the heat was doubled, they died. By purely chemical analysis, the proteins still appeared to have the same properties. Yet in biological tests, the heated substance would no longer support life. The conclusion was that animals couldn't obtain optimal protein supply from thoroughly cooked muscle meats, as was previously taught, but that uncooked vegetable nutrients supplemented with whole grains and cereals can do this. Milk proteins likewise suffer decisive damage from cooking and pasteurization processes.

To summarize, it is clear that there is no important difference between the diet necessary for optimal health and the diet necessary for best performance in athletics. Although it is not possible in this short article to give details of a modern full-value diet, I can list general guidelines.

- The diet should consist, as much as possible, of only full-valued foods. I advise complete avoidance of manufactured nutrients. This means renouncing refined flour and sugar, and chemically extracted fats.
- Eat fruits and vegetables in raw form. The greater the share of raw products, the greater will be a person's performance capacity.
- Fill the protein needs with nuts, soybeans, whole grains, and cereals, without relying on muscle meats.
- Drink only raw (unpasteurized) milk.
- Use only butter, cream, and cold-pressed oils (such as wheat-germ oil) to fulfill fat needs.

It is important to recognize that health and performance capacity rest on several pillars. No single one contributes sufficiently without the others. Mastery of life's problems through harmony in the mental-spiritual realm is just as meaningful as whole-value, natural nutrition, sufficient physical movement, and abstention from various foods. Only by a meaningful union of all of these can a person be truly healthy.

4
The Return to Nature

Nutritional theory seems to be moving backward. "New" nutritional thinking—all the talk about natural foods—isn't actually new at all. For only a heartbeat in the span of time has man been eating prepared and preserved, refined and rejuvenated foods. Only a few decades of this kind of eating has convinced many nutritionists that this is the wrong way to go—that man must get back to simpler, fresher food sources or pay a high penalty.

Food dies. Every step it moves up the preparation ladder, away from its fresh and raw form, it surrenders a bit of its life—until finally it is empty and dead. Eating empty, dead food is worse than useless, according to new nutritionists such as Dr. Brucker. Brucker basically reflects the thinking of Are Waerland, a Swede of Finnish birth, who popularized the Waerland dietary system in Europe. His methods center on eating foods as close to their natural state as possible. (See chapter 1 for details on the Waerland system.)

European runners follow the Waerland program in fairly large numbers. Some have had notable success, particularly in being able to run well year after year, in the best of physical health.

Erik Ostbye, a Swede, is now over 50 years old. He still runs the marathon under 2:30, and is one of his country's leading runners a dozen years after winning his first national championship. In 1943, Ostbye was suffering from a severe intestinal disorder. A switch to the Waerland diet cured him. He has stayed with this dietary plan—with a few individual variations—to this day. Diet is the decisive factor in his running, he says. He doesn't think a person on a "normal" diet could accomplish the things he does after more than two decades of hard training.

The case of John Systad, a Norwegian, is similar. Though Systad was never as good a marathoner as Ostbye, he labored under greater handicaps. Systad suffered with asthma as a child. When he was 12 years old, a severe inflammation in both lungs and an extremely high fever threatened his life. He pulled through, but with a drastically reduced breathing capacity that weakened him generally. Systad's mother switched him to a raw-foods diet. As he got stronger, he added long hikes, sunbathing, and fasting to his health-building routine. By the time he was 18, Systad was strong enough to compete in 30-kilometer walks. Then, after World War II, he switched to distance running. He was already 34 years old when he started. Systad eventually won eight Norwegian championships—five in the marathon. The last victory came at age 43.

Systad became convinced that since fruit gave him great energy, it must be possible to live almost exclusively on fruit. He followed this basic diet:

Early morning: pure orange or grapefruit juice

Breakfast: herb tea and sometimes an apple

Mid-morning: fruit

Evening: only "meal" of the day, consisting of many onions, a raw and a cooked potato, and two slices of whole-grain bread

The Dutch marathon record-holder, Aad Steylen, follows the same sort of diet, though less severe than Systad's. Steylen ran a 2:19 marathon several years ago at the age of 33. "I am convinced," he says, "that through a particular kind of diet, combined with optimal training, one does remain in top form for many years longer without exhausting the body."

Steylan recalls his own dietary experience:

> In 1961, I began to change my nutrition to a natural diet with raw vegetables, salads, rice, whole cereals, fruit. Then in 1963 I became a vegetarian. I now nourish myself with whole cereals, rice, raw vegetables, salads, fruit, potatoes, whole wheat, millet, various herbs, whole-grain bread, curds, sour milk, nuts, herb teas, and cold-pressed vegetable oils (such as wheat-germ oil, which I consider important for its vitamin E content).
>
> On the basis of this diet, combined with my training, I have been able to attain the best successes. My experiences showed me that one has a

more consistent performance development through the season with this natural nutrition, and is protected against colds and related troubles. Since beginning this diet, I have had hardly any infectious diseases, tendon, cartilage, joint, or muscle injuries. I trace this back to my natural diet, which provides the body with the necessary nutritional and building substances. Nutrients are supposed to give vital energy. They are just as important as training, and can be the foundation of health.

5
A Good Diet? Try It

Stephen Streeter

Competitive runners are constantly searching for tools to improve their racing. Unfortunately, while there has been great advancement in training techniques over the past few decades, there still appears to be no consensus on what constitutes the proper diet for the runner. Since the experts often don't agree on this controversial subject, we are often led to believe it doesn't matter what we eat.

I decided to challenge the idea that diet is irrelevant to athletic performance, as well as the claim that individual differences prevent the formation of general principles. So I experimented with one of the theoretically designed diet systems of a nutritional expert. I thought it was important to adhere to the proposed system quite religiously, since this would be the only fair test of its effects on my running.

After researching the literature on diet, I found the most sensible approach seemed to be "natural hygiene," as advocated by Herbert Shelton. Natural hygiene is based on the premise that disease is caused by improper nutrition, and that true health can be restored by only governing one's living habits by "natural laws." These natural laws have formed along with the evolution of the human body, and thus are based on biology and human physiology.

To see how this ties in with running, it helps to examine the hygienic concept of health. Health is a broad term we use to describe an individual's physical and mental well-being, usually implying freedom from disease. It is based not only on diet, but also exercise, rest, and one's general environment. This dependence of nutrition on many interacting factors is the reason diet has been a difficult area for scientists to study.

This is also why good health can lead to improved running performances. If we are in a superior state of health, we can train harder and withstand a greater amount of stress than if we devote energy to fighting nutritional deficiencies. I felt that as a knowledgeable runner I was meeting all the requirements for good health as far as exercise and rest were concerned. Now I was in a position to determine the importance of a proper diet.

Shelton's recommended diet is really quite simple, consisting of fresh fruits, vegetables, and nuts. The science of food-combining, while ignored by many nutritionists, plays an important role in the hygienic diet. It is based on the physiology of the human digestive system, and is designed to assure maximum assimilation of life-sustaining nutrients.

At first, I was overwhelmed at the apparent complexity of rules concerning acceptable combinations. But I soon learned how to classify foods by their chemical compositions, which made it easier to plan than if I were following strict menus.

Breakfast consisted solely of fruit, since this was quickly digested and gave one a good source of energy to start the day. Lunch was a starch meal, usually whole-grain bread or a starchy vegetable like potatoes or rice, and was accompanied by a large raw salad of greens. Dinner was the protein meal, provided either by nuts or certain vegetables (corn, for example) and sometimes cheese. In addition, the usual salad of succulent vegetables was prepared with no dressings, oils, or spices.

I followed this basic pattern of eating for several months while training moderately in preparation for the cross-country season. I must admit that the elimination of all condiments, such as salt and pepper, as well as refined commercial products, was not an easy adjustment, particularly since I was raised on conventional American foods like hamburgers, hot dogs, ice cream, and so on. This adjustment was difficult, since these foods stimulate the nervous system. When you suddenly cut off the course of stimulation, you are bound to feel withdrawal symptoms. However, I found that Shelton was right when he advised not to taper off, but to make the radical change and try to adjust. This is the best way to prevent slipping back into the cycle of stimulation, followed by a period of withdrawal and the need for the stimulant all over again. The diet is not really as bland as it sounds, and I found that after several months my senses were much more finely attuned to the delicate flavors of unseasoned vegetables and fresh fruit.

The first and most noticeable result I experienced after switching my diet was a marked reduction in body weight. This is a clear advantage for runners who tend to put on weight easily. Since many runners are already light (as I was), this reduction probably wouldn't be as helpful. Yet even I could feel a better tolerance to heat, as well as a greater sense of mobility in my running style.

One of the reasons for this is the replacement of high-calorie foods such as cakes and pies with foods of a higher fiber content, and consequently less refined starches. Perhaps even more important is the impossibility of overeating, at least without being acutely aware of it. I found that my appetite was a much better gauge of how much food I could comfortably digest, although I never left the table feeling unsatiated.

I also learned from the principles of natural hygiene that it is better to reduce food intake during times of stress. In the runner's case, this means eating less before and after races. Following this advice, I found that the recovery period after a hard race was generally shorter and easier to tolerate.

It used to be that I practically had to force myself to eat after racing, thinking I had to replenish those exhausted reserves. While it is true that one loses many nutrients during the course of a long race, it does no good to stuff oneself with food if the digestive system is still trying to recover from the stress of heavy exercise. Thus, I found it was better to wait until hunger returned, signaling that the body was ready to perform the necessary digestive processes that enable it to replace appropriate nutrients.

A third result I attribute to the hygienic diet was an increased resistance to sickness. I never even had anything resembling a cold, and I seemed able to withstand all kinds of environmental stresses without any ill-effects. It probably isn't fair to draw this conclusion based on such a short trial period, but I mention it only because I really felt I was experiencing an improved state of health. Perhaps this was the "high" that so many natural living advocates are always talking about.

In general, then, the changes I experienced after switching to a hygienic diet, while not staggering, were significant in providing a more pleasant atmosphere in which to train and race. While training still plays the predominant role in good racing times, I believe that proper nutrition (including some type of natural foods diet) provides the runner with the best foundation for withstanding a heavier stress load.

Maybe Herbert Shelton and the natural hygienists don't have all the answers. But it's unfortunate more people aren't willing to test their ideas. It was incredible to me the amount of resistance I encountered from friends and family when I refused to eat "normally." Although being a runner made me somewhat used to this sort of reaction, I found it difficult at times to escape the stigma of fanaticism, merely because I wanted to test a nutritional theory. While running is usually done in isolation or with fellow runners, eating plays a large social role in a society that demands conformity.

My experiment convinced me it's about time that runners who use the activity as an excuse to eat anything and everything step back and take a long look at the effect of their diet on their health and consequently their running. It was Pythagoras who said, "Choose what is best; habit will soon render it agreeable and easy." To decide what is best, we need to study the experiences of people who aren't afraid to break out of the dietary rut.

6
Internal Disturbances

In the hair-splitting world of running, where good and bad performances are divided by seconds and tenth-seconds, the effects of sound nutrition are subtle. The worth of a beneficial diet can't be measured strictly by the stopwatch. A runner can have an ideal diet and still not notice dramatic improvements in time. The body works that way; when it's working best, it's noticed least. It's said you don't really appreciate the water until the well runs dry. And you don't appreciate how important nutrition is until something goes wrong inside. Then the effects are dramatic. These you *can* measure.

Chapters 2 and 3 centered on sound general nutrition. These factors have a rather indirect role in performance. By promoting good overall health, they create an environment in which runners can train to their maximum. But no matter how good their eating habits are, runners progress little without the training. The quantity and quality of running makes differences of seconds and tenths.

Here, we're talking about the direct influence of diet. Unfortunately, it's usually a negative one. No matter how well the training has gone, dietary miscalculations can spoil everything.

Runners operate under physical and sometimes emotional stress. Dr. George Sheehan calls the runner "man at his maximum." Stress situations make runners peculiarly susceptible to diet-related irregularities that don't often strike people who operate on a lower plane. Trouble pops up at the worst possible times, when stress is highest, usually when there's a race to run. The common symptoms are internal upsets, which cause vomiting or diarrhea, and stomach or intestinal pains, which destroy running rhythm.

There appear to be two main causes of severe internal distress:

Eating too much too soon before running. Prerace diet is such a ritual that it prompted Arthur Lydiard to observe, "The way runners eat before races, you'd think they were worried about dying of malnutrition after 50 meters." Dr. Ernst van Aaken, a German scientist and coach, says runners are wise not to eat *anything* before competition. According to him, the body is perfectly capable of "living off its own resources" during the race, and every ounce of food increases the system's burden. The system is already busy enough, van Aaken says, and extra food only increases the chance of trouble.

Eating the wrong foods at the wrong times. Certain stomachs can't tolerate certain food groups, and they react violently to them—particularly in tense situations. Dr. Sheehan listed these foods in his booklet *Encyclopedia of Athletic Medicine.* Surprisingly, he started his list with two "perfect" foods: milk and bread (or more correctly, all grain products containing the substance gluten).

Other suspect foods are:

1. The highly allergenic ones (chocolate, shellfish, strawberries, pork, melon, nuts, citrus fruits, egg white) "cause stomach pains, diarrhea, bloating, rash, itching, head aches, nasal stuffiness, migraine headaches, etc."

2. Excessive roughage (raw fruit, raw vegetables, nuts, corn, beer, baked beans, cabbage, etc.) "cause[s] gas, bloating, pain, thin cigar-like stools in runners with spastic colons."

3. Coffee "causes hyperacidity and stomach spasm in some people."

The problem with milk is that some people literally can't stand it. Their bodies aren't equipped to handle it. Dr. Sheehan has written, "Milk, after the second decade of life is something most Greek Cypriots, Arabs, Ashkenazi Jews and American Negroes should shun. These people from traditional non-milking areas (and this includes among others the Bantu, Chinese, Thai, Greenland Eskimo and Peruvian Indian) can have bloating, gas and stomach pains, along with loud noises, after even the small amounts of milk used in cooking." Dr. Theodore Bayless of Johns Hopkins University, an expert on the milk intolerance problem, says about 8 percent of Caucasians also have trouble handling milk. He says this is because they have a deficency of the enzyme that digests lactose, a sugar in milk. Sheehan adds that "most people with milk allergy do not drink milk anyway through some body intuition. If you have never been much of a milk drinker, I think you should accept this "body wisdom" and seek the necessary protein, calcium and vitamins A and D in some other foods or supplements."

Bread and most other grain-based foods also present problems for some runners. Sheehan says, "Many men, it appears, cannot live by bread *at all*, much less alone." He cites the case study of one of his patients, a distance runner named Gary Berthiaume.

"Every time he entered a long, tough race," Dr. Sheehan writes, "he came down with severe stomach pain. Sometimes he would have diarrhea and blood as well. When not running and at all other times, he had little or no bowel complaints."

When Gary sought help from another doctor, he was told nothing was abnormal and that his difficulties stemmed from "too much stress during the race and too much nervousness anticipating it." Berthiaume already knew that. But telling a distance runner to avoid stress is like telling a swimmer not to get wet.

Sheehan continues:

> Stress obviously played a part. He only developed symptoms after a hard run. But he was peculiarly susceptible to these abdominal complaints, and no one knew why.... He had no known allergies, and even varying the pre-race meal didn't help. He continued to experience pain severe enough to double him up soon after the race was over. He finally reduced his pre-race feeding to bread and milk, but he still had trouble. There, as it turned out, lay the answer.
>
> Bread, or more specifically gluten—protein found in all grains except corn and rice—was his difficulty. In its full-blown state the inability to handle gluten is called "sprue," meaning chronic diarrhea. It now appears that some of us may have sprue. Most don't, but many, when placed under stress, can become symptomatic. When the rat-race pushes us too fast or too far, our bowels will let us know. Gluten is always there in our diet, in the bread and baked goods, in the cereals and cereal products, and hidden in soups and gravies, ice cream, wheat germ, mayonnaise and even beer and ale.

The ironic thing in this, Sheehan points out, is that milk

and bread—long considered the perfect foods for stomach disorders—have turned out to be major causes of the ailments they were supposed to cure.

Part II
The Body's Fuel

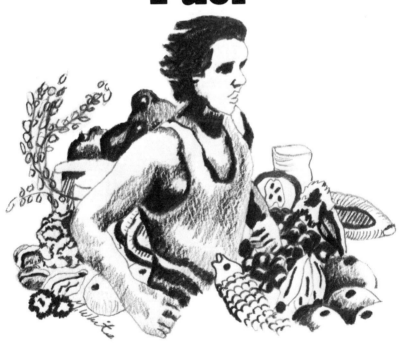

7
Two Sources of Energy

M. E. Houston

To run continuously at a fast pace, a runner requires oxygen and fuel as the essential components for performance. The cardiorespiratory system, which is improved by training, transports the oxygen to the working muscles. Efficient delivery of oxygen is a prime requirement for distance-running success. However, the fuel with which the oxygen combines is also very important.

There are three fuels available to all cells: protein, carbohydrate, and fat. It is a well-established fact that protein is not used as a fuel to any significant extent when the caloric content of the diet is adequate. Hence, fat and carbohydrate are the chief substances employed in the daily energy production cycles.

If we look solely at energy content, fat is a better fuel than carbohydrate. Each gram of fat yields 9.3 calories; each gram of carbohydrate produces 4.1 calories. All of us contain stored energy sufficient to run tremendous distances. However, our speed of running is limited by how rapidly we convey the oxygen to the working muscles.

It is important, therefore, to focus attention on fuel efficiency. The question is, then, which produces more energy per given amount of oxygen—carbohydrate or fat? Each gram of fat produces 4.5 calories of energy for every liter of oxygen, whereas carbohydrate produces 5.0 calories per liter of oxygen. Thus, if we are limited by the amount of oxygen at the muscle cell level, it would be better to burn carbohydrate than fat as fuel.

Each of us, even the leanest runner, has enough stored fat to run at least 100 miles were we able to get it to the working muscle cells. But carbohydrate is not stored to any large extent in the body. There are three areas where carbohydrate is stored: (1) in the bloodstream as blood glucose; (2) in the liver as liver glycogen; and (3) as muscle glycogen.

Blood glucose is controlled in the body so that a certain minimum level is always present. The liver (the organ that stores the glucose as glycogen) maintains the blood glucose levels at the minimum concentration. Since the blood glucose concentration is so essential and since the liver acts as a reservoir for glucose, then the muscle glycogen depots are filled only when blood and liver stores are adequate. Furthermore, studies have revealed that blood glucose is not employed to any appreciable extent as a fuel by the muscles during work. This underscores the need for adequate stores of muscle glycogen.

A peculiar situation exists in the body. Fat may be produced from carbohydrate, excess protein, and dietary fat. However, neither fat nor protein can produce carbohydrate to any appreciable extent. Hence, only dietary carbohydrate may act as the source of muscle glycogen.

It has been discovered that endurance athletes have larger than normal muscle glycogen depots in the muscles utilized by the activity. Thus, a marathoner has more glycogen stored in his leg muscles than a nonrunner of the same size. However, they might have the same amount in the shoulder muscles, since these are not the essential working muscles for a distance runner.

There are rather large differences in muscle glycogen concentration throughout the body. But unlike stores of many other substances, glycogen cannot be moved from muscle to muscle. It is, in essence, locked into the particular muscle where it was formed.

During the past five years, some remarkable studies have been performed on the working muscles of man. Many of these studies have shown a definite relationship between the ability to perform long-endurance work and the stores of muscle glycogen. That is, subjects were able to work much longer at a high work load if their muscle glycogen depots were filled than if these depots were only partially filled. Furthermore, when the glycogen in the muscles was depleted, the subjects were exhausted. Further work was possible only if the work load was decreased.

Since the carbohydrate content of the diet profoundly influences the amount of muscle glycogen, it appears that a high-carbohydrate diet is necessary in sporting events where large quantities of glycogen are employed. Such a situation occurs in distance running, cross-country skiing, and long-distance bicycle racing. A high-carbohydrate diet plus endurance training results in larger-than-average glycogen depots in athletes. Furthermore, there is a special diet that can increase muscle glycogen levels to super values. This special diet requires one week, and is therefore suited for the big race:

1. One week before the race, the glycogen supplies in the working muscles are depleted by a long run—about the same distance as the event itself, though slower.

2. For the next three days, a diet devoid of carbohydrate is consumed. This means that the food eaten will be fat and protein (meat, eggs, fish, cottage cheese, cabbage, celery, lettuce, tomatoes, cheeses). As a result, the glycogen in muscles, depleted by the practice distance, is kept low. Training is more difficult here since fat will be the primary training fuel. (But training before big events generally is reduced, anyway).

3. The last three days before the race, a high carbohydrate diet is eaten. This means supplementing the regular diet with carbohydrate-rich foods: bread, potatoes, vegetables (beans, peas, sweet potatoes), spaghetti, etc. It should be emphasized that gorging is not the idea; one is merely shifting the food balance to those foods supplying carbohydrate.

4. On race day, nothing special need be eaten. As usual, the runner should eat lightly beforehand, and only those foods that agree with him.

The benefits of this prerace diet have been confirmed by Swedish physiologist Bengt Saltin. Two groups of physically fit students ran two 30-kilometer races, three weeks apart. For each race, either the special diet or a normal mixed meal was eaten. The result was that performances averaged eight minutes faster when the experimental subjects ate the special diet. This should have tremendous significance to the seasoned runner, where seconds alone can separate the top finishers and can result in personal records.

It is evident from these findings that carbohydrates are quite important in the diet of distance runners—not only before races but while in heavy training. Runners should be careful to maintain high-carbohydrate intake at a time when the percentage of this element in the American diet is decreasing.

8
Prerace Eating Plan

If any one man could claim credit for turning runners away from steak and eggs and turning them on to spaghetti and cookies, it is Per-Olof Astrand. Astrand, a Swedish medical doctor, is an avid cross-country skier. Since the demands of cross-country skiing are much like distance running, he has more than an academic interest in the diet and performance of endurance athletes. Astrand has experimented extensively, and his work has been well publicized.

Several years ago, Astrand wrote a long article for the magazine *Nutrition Today*. It summarized his then-revolutionary findings. He made two claims, which at the time were startling. Now they are common knowledge.

- Protein foods play no immediate part in the energy production of exercising athletes.
- Energy comes from a judicious mixture of carbohydrate and fats. Proper dosage can increase stamina by 300 percent.

Astrand had the facts to back up his statements. First, the matter of protein:

> In 1866, two German scientists, Pettenkofer and Voit, showed that combustion of protein was no higher during heavy exercise than during rest. Since these century-old studies, these findings have been frequently confirmed.... In one experiment, we compared cross-country skiers who raced 20-50 miles in one day with resting athletes used as controls. There was no noticeable difference in the amount of protein used.
>
> There seems no doubt that it is proper to exclude protein from consideration as a fuel for working muscle cells.

Carbohydrates and fats are the fuels, he says. He learned that fat is the main fuel supply in mild exercise.

He takes an example from his own distance skiing experience:

We participated in a ski tour in the mountains. During three days, we covered a distance of about 65 kilometers (39 miles). The calculated caloric output was a total of some 18,000 calories. Only 1,000 calories were supplied. These came almost exclusively in the form of carbohydrate. Some 14,000-15,000 calories were probably derived from fat (stored in the body). With the few calories in the form of sugar taken at appropriate intervals and by avoiding peak loads, the three days of heavy work could be completed. We experienced the symptoms of hypoglycemia (low blood-sugar) on only a few occasions during the test.

As exercise becomes more intense, however, carbohydrate assumes prime importance. According to Astrand, "The utilization of carbohydrate depends on the oxygen supplied to the working muscles. The more inadequate the oxygen supply, the higher the carbohydrate utilization." This would be the case in most running events, which are relatively short and fast, and have a degree of oxygen debt involved.

So the obvious way to increase available energy for running is to increase the amount of carbohydrate in the diet. It is a physiological fact, though, that carbohydrate—converted to glycogen—is in relatively short supply in the body. It can't be stored easily and increased indefinitely. There are limits. And to reach even these, Astrand says, requires careful dietary control. But with the kind of control he recommends, the results can be astounding.

Here's how he says to go about building available energy reserves:

> The proper preparation for a competition in any endurance event exceeding 30-60 minutes would be to exercise to exhaustion the same muscles that will be used in the event. This should be done about one week in advance to exhaust glycogen stores. Then the diet should be almost exclusively fat and protein for about three days. This keeps the glycogen content of the exercising muscles low. As the big day nears, the athlete should add large quantities of carbohydrates. *Add* is the word, because the intake of fats and protein should be continued. This regimen is recommended for anyone preparing himself for prolonged, severe exercise. We have found it works.

The Swedish doctor offers laboratory evidence that it works. Several of his collegues tested 20 subjects, who rode to exhaustion on a stationary bicycle. Before their rides, the athletes were checked for muscle glycogen content in their upper legs (the hardest working muscles in this test).

They followed a normal "mixed" diet. The average glycogen count was 1.6 grams per 100 grams of muscle. The exhausted riders stopped after 90 minutes. The glycogen level had dropped to 0.1 g./100 g. "With the glycogen depots emptied," Astrand says, "the work has to cease, or the subject has to reduce the rate of work."

Astrand's own tests supported these findings. He tested nine subjects, who worked on the bicycle at about the same intensity as those above. Astrand, however, took his subjects through four different rides—each on a different dietary routine.

A "mixed" diet. (Three days.) The starting glycogen content was 1.75 grams per 100 grams of muscle. The average ride was 114 minutes.

All all-protein and fat diet. (Three days.) Initial muscle glycogen level was only 0.63 grams per 100—or about a third the mixed diet amount. The riders could only go half as far as before—or 57 minutes.

A carbohydrate-rich diet. (Three days.) Starting glycogen levels climbed to 3.51 grams—twice as high as with the mixed diet. The subjects lasted 167 minutes on the bicycle—or about 50% more than they had on a mixed diet.

A "seven-day-diet plan." Astrand says, "The most pronounced effect was obtained if the glycogen content was first emptied by heavy prolonged exercise and a diet very rich in carbohydrates given for (the last) three days. With this procedure, the glycogen content could exceed 4.0 grams per 100 grams wet muscle, and the heavy work tolerated for prolonged periods—sometimes more than four hours (240 minutes)."

Riding at a steady rate, the test subjects increased their "distances" by 200 to 400 percent—simply by changing what they ate. This study shows that dietary adjustments can improve endurance—the ability to hold a fixed pace longer before getting exhausted. It isn't clear what the adjustment means to people trying to run a fixed distance faster.

9
Going Beyond Theory

Laboratory studies are valuable. They have control and precision not found on the tracks and roads. Yet there is an air of unreality about them. Both the methods and the results can go over an unscientific runner's head, and leave him with little understanding of the practical significance of the lab work.

Scientifically, perhaps timed running tests are less accurate than those in the laboratory. But no doubt they hit a more responsive note with everyday runners. Swedish physiologists J. Karlsson and B. Saltin have made such a dietary study that runners can really get their teeth into. The results spell out what carbohydrate-loading can mean in terms of time improvement. Karlsson and Saltin tested 10 trained distance runners. They ran two 30-kilometer races, with three weeks of recovery in between. Running conditions for the two tests were as identical as possible. However, there was a difference in what the runners ate the week before each event.

Before the first 30-kilometer test, half of the subjects ate a normal mixed diet, while the other half overloaded with carbohydrates. In the second test, the two groups were reversed. The prerun program involved at least a two-hour run one week before the test, followed by three days of low-carbohydrate regimen while continuing training. That was followed by high-carbohydrate intake for three days with no heavy work.

The results of the two tests were combined. The "normal-diet" runners averaged 2:23:00 for the 30-kilometer runs. The "carbohydrate-loaded" individuals ran 2:15:18 on the average. In other words, the per-man improvement amounted to over 7½ minutes, 5½ percent, or 25 seconds per mile. Any way you look at it, the effect of adjusted food intake was startling in this case.

The 10 runners were tested for muscle glycogen levels before and after each run. On high-carbohydrate diets, the runners had about twice the stored glycogen that they had on normal mixed diets. The prerun figures were 3.52 grams per 100 grams of tissue for the former and 1.77 for the latter. During the runs, the subjects lost more glycogen after a carbohydrate-loading diet than after a normal one—but they had much more to lose. The postrun figures were 1.90 grams per 100 in the first case and 0.52 in the second. Even after the high-carbohydrate run, glycogen levels were higher than normal. The significance of this is that glycogen supplies energy for the working muscles. As long as glycogen levels stay high, muscles can keep working at a steady pace. When glycogen is depleted, work must slow or stop.

In this test, Karlsson and Saltin recorded split times at several points in the 30-kilometer runs. They found that runners on the high-carbohydrate routine maintained a higher pace in the last two-thirds of the run than when they were on mixed diets. Times for the first third of the run were about equal, regardless of what they ate. However, on mixed diets severe glycogen depletion set in after 10 kilometers. To the man, the runners lost time from then on—in some cases more than 15 minutes compared with their carbohydrate-loaded performances.

10
Diet in Distance Runs
Dr. Enrico Arcelli

In perhaps no other athletic event is fundamental knowlege of physiology of such great practical value as in a long-distance run such as the marathon. Athletes who are aware of the physical demands of distance running are better able to prevent crises in competition. These include dehydration, hyperthermia (excessive body heat), hypoglycemia (low blood sugar), and exhaustion of the glycogen stores in muscle tissues. All are related to nutrition, and I'll deal with them here. The material is subdivided for quick reference, but in fact many of the subjects are interrelated.

The caloric cost of running. For every kilometer run at race tempo, the marathon runner uses about 0.9 calorie per kilogram of body weight. A well-conditioned athlete may get by on less (e.g., 0.8 calorie) while a person not accustomed to running may supply about 1.0 calorie. For the entire marathon distance (42.2 kilometers), an athlete weighing 60 kilograms and running at a cost of 0.9 cal./kg. x km. will have to expend about 2,280 calories. He uses about 55 calories per kilometer. For the same well-trained runner, the per-mile caloric cost converts to about 88. He uses 0.66 calorie per pound for every mile at racing pace. The cost per pound for each kilometer is 0.4.

Dehydration and salt deficit. During a marathon run in mild weather, the runner loses an average of two or three liters of sweat (about four to six pounds). In great heat, some runners lose five or more liters, and in extreme cases even 10 percent of their body weight. A loss of this magnitude can put a runner in a dehydration crisis state. It is therefore important that the runner go to the starting line well hydrated, and that he replace at least part of the water lost in sweat during the race. Above all, it is advisable for the runner under conditions of great heat to drink at least enough to quench his thirst. It must also be pointed out that perspiration contains 0.2 to 0.5 percent salt. When the organism is in such a state of salt deficiency, perspiration can become difficult. Some authorities take the view that one should add salt to the drinks taken during the run. The salt balance is thus maintained, and the time the drink spends in the stomach is decreased.

Water of hydration and water of oxidation. During a marathon run, 2.7 grams of water are freed for every gram of burned glycogen—which is bound to the water as "water of hydration." An athlete following the preparatory diet (described below) uses about 375 grams of glycogen during the marathon; about 1,000 grams of water are freed during the process. After a mixed diet, the glycogen use drops to about 280 grams, bound with 750 grams of water. After a fat-protein diet, the glycogen consumption amounts to only about 185 grams, bound with 500 grams of water.

Aside from this, about 300 grams of "water of oxidation" are freed during the burning of glycogen and fatty acids. In all, between 800 and 1,300 grams of water of hydration and oxidation can be removed from the body in the form of sweat—without the blood or other tissues having to give it up. This is one of the reasons why marathon runners may lose more than 8 percent of their body weight as sweat during the run, and yet show no symptoms of dehydration—at least not to the extent that would be seen in someone who loses the same amount of sweat without muscular work. The significance of this profuse sweating is that it acts as a coolant during the race. Dietary control can influence the perspiration rate.

Glycogen and fatty acids. Glycogen and fatty acids are the fuels from which the energy for the muscles comes. Glycogen is already in the muscles in tiny mass particles. Fatty acids, on the other hand, come from the stores of fat and arrive at the muscles via the blood. Before the start of a marathon, there are about 100 grams of glycogen in the muscles. At the finish, this amount is severely reduced. Fatty acids stored in fat deposits make up about 2 to 3 percent of the body weight (about 1.5 kilograms in a runner weighing 60 kilograms).

Significance of a carbohydrate-rich diet. In 1939, Christiansen and Hansen found that physical work of a given intensity can be continued for an average of four hours when an athlete has eaten predominantly carbohydrates; two hours with a mixed diet; and less than 1½ hours with a fat-protein diet. Recently, other Scandinavians determined that a carbohydrate-rich diet increases the glycogen content of the muscles, and that this high-glycogen content permits more stress at a given intensity (or, if one speaks of a race at a fixed distance such as the marathon, that less time is needed to run the distance).

Maximum glycogen content of the muscles. For an athlete eating a mixed diet, the glycogen content of the muscles is about 1.5 grams per 100 grams of muscle. After a longer-than-normal period of stress in training, this glycogen content sinks significantly.

If the athlete then eats predominantly carbohydrate-rich meals, the glycogen content of the muscles rises sharply after only a few meals. By the third day, values of over three grams per 100 grams of muscle can be attained. This is twice the normal glycogen content.

If, on the other hand, a pure fat-protein diet is maintained after decreasing the glycogen content by training—and no carbohydrates are eaten—only a very small amount of glycogen is maintained in the muscles. Such a diet has no immediate usefulness, but is important in creating a "sugar hunger" in the muscles. If the athlete then eats carbohydrates exclusively for the next three days, the glycogen content of the muscles reaches about four grams per 100 grams of muscle (and in certain cases even over five grams—or more than three times the normal value).

Therefore, if the marathon runner wants to go to the start with a high glycogen content in the muscles, he should, beginning six days before the competition: (1) take a long training session, (2) maintain a fat-protein diet for three days, and (3) then follow a high-carbohydrate diet for the final three days.

Training during the "preparatory diet." Suppose that the marathon will be on a Sunday. The last long training run takes place on the previous Sunday. From then until Wednesday the athlete stays on a fat-protein diet and trains over very limited distances. The lack of glycogen will make training very tiring. Thursday, Friday, and Saturday there should be little or no training, in order to promote the storing of glycogen. On race day, the athlete will eat lightly, if at all—depending on the starting time of the race. If there is a long time between the last meal and competition, he may take sugar in solid or dissolved form 15-30 minutes before the start.

If a runner cannot follow the preparatory diet completely, he should nevertheless do this partially—even though the advantage is not as great. Above all, the last four to six meals should consist solely of carbohydrates. This diet should begin after a lengthy training session, and there should be very little training during the dietary period.

Weight gain from "preparatory diet." The athlete following a preparatory diet will go to the starting line weighing several hundred grams more than one who has been on a mixed diet. If this weight increase is one kilogram (2.2 pounds), the runner will have to use about 1.6 percent more energy during the first stage of the race. However, this runner will also lose weight faster than one who has been eating a mixed diet during the week before the race. There is also less need to drink.

The increase in weight is attributable less to storage of glycogen than to the fact that this occurs in hydrated form. Each gram of glucose corresponds to about 2.7 grams of water of hydration.

Advantages of "preparatory diet." The athlete has a better "breathing quotient." In other words, he can produce 4.92 calories of energy for every liter of oxygen after a carbohydrate-rich diet—compared to 4.86 calories after a mixed diet, and 4.80 calories after a fat-rich diet. Compared with a mixed diet, then, the energy advantage of an "excess glucose" diet amounts to about 1.2 percent. However, we also saw that weight gain amounts to 1.6 percent or more. The disadvantage due to additional weight seems to neutralize the benefit of extra energy.

In reality, though, one must also consider the following:

1. The athlete who has followed the preparatory diet loses added weight quickly.

2. Runners on a preparatory diet will not run the risk of glycogen deficiency crisis. Glycogen will still be present in sufficient amounts during the last kilometers of the marathon.
3. Athletes store greater amounts of water during a preparatory diet, and run less risk of dehydration or heat-crisis.
4. The glycogen stores of the liver also increase. Since the liver regulates the glucose content of the blood, a hypoglycemia crisis is easily avoided in this way.

Sugar eaten during competiton. Going to the starting line with muscles heavily enriched with glycogen undoubtedly is an advantage for the marathoner. Can one achieve the same advantage by eating sugar during the run? The answer is clearly no. Aside from the difficulty of eating the same amount of sugar during a run as we spoke of concerning the preparatory diet, physiological factors argue against this. Normally, sugar (and all carbohydrates) are converted to monosaccharides during digestion and are carried into the circulatory system. These are transferred to the cells with the help of a hormone—insulin. During physical exertion, the insulin level sinks, and the monosaccharides can no longer be transferred to the muscles. Sugar intake is somewhat useful during the run, but less as a source of glycogen for muscles than to maintain the blood sugar balance.

Blood glucose content. Normally, 100 grams of blood contains about one gram of glucose (1 g. percent). If this amount sinks to 0.8 g. percent or less, we have hypoglycemia (a deficiency of glucose). A glucose deficiency leads to severe disturbances and, if the glucose falls to less than 0.5 g. percent, even unconsciousness.

The glucose content of the blood is usually maintained at a normal level by glucose present in the liver—in the form of glycogen. If at the start of a marathon the glycogen stores in the liver of a runner are insufficient, the runner risks a hypoglycemia crisis during the run. As mentioned in the previous section, eating sugar during the run can help the runner somewhat, but not nearly as much as if he had followed the full preparatory diet.

We have found that marathon runners who prepared in the

way outlined here arrived fresher at the finish line. These runners confirmed that they had suffered less than in runs without this preparation. The usefulness of the preparatory diet is therefore beyond doubt, even aside from its time advantages.

11
The Vital Role of Glucose
M. H. M. Arnold

One of the most remarkable things about the human body is its flexibility of performance. The same person—the same body—can dash for 100 yards, run a marathon, or walk the length of England. Although much the same muscles are used in all three cases, the rate at which work is done and the duration of effort vary enormously.

The long-distance walker will consume energy at the rate of 350 calories an hour intermittently for around 200 hours. The marathon runner uses about 900 calories an hour for over two hours. The sprinter burns energy at the rate of about 10,000 calories an hour, but only for a few seconds. A high jumper will work at the fantastic rate of 100,000 calories an hour, for a fraction of a second. Because the range is so broad, it is reasonable to suspect that different energy supply mechanisms are involved. This is in fact the case.

The "single-effort" athlete—jumper or thrower—obtains his burst of energy from the almost explosive breakdown of a substance called adenosine triphosphate within the muscles. Skill in these activities depends largely on triggering this supply of energy at just the right moment. The performer also builds up an extra energy supply in the form of momentum from a run or a spin.

The sprinter simply runs as fast as his legs will carry him. He gets his energy from the glycogen in his muscles. His body demands six liters of oxygen during a 10-second dash. This he cannot get, because the most his heart and lungs can supply in that short time is a liter. The body goes into debt for oxygen, obtaining energy by converting glycogen into lactic acid without the use of oxygen. In fact, during a sprint the lungs have little to do, and a sprinter can run 100 yards while holding his breath. When the race is over, the sprinter pants. He is repaying the debt by converting lactic acid back into glycogen. The oxygen debt process is extravagant. In 10 seconds, about a half-pound of glycogen is used up. True, all but about a quarter of an ounce is paid back later, but the whole half-pound must be there to start with. The glycogen stores of the body must be adequate to meet the demand.

There is a limit to the oxygen debt that can be incurred. This is set by the increasing muscular discomfort as lactic acid levels build up in the blood. The longest distance than can be run at full speed is about 300 yards. At longer distances, a runner must take care not to get into oxygen debt too soon. However, beyond the mile oxygen debt declines progressively in significance and is replaced by the factor of energy supply.

The maximum rate at which oxygen can be supplied continuously for prolonged periods (without incurring oxygen debt) is about 2.5 liters per minute. This is the so-called steady state at which energy is being used up at the rate of about 800 calories per hour. This corresponds to a speed of 6-7 m.p.h., and to a glycogen usage of around 200 grams (about a half-pound) per hour.

The total stock of glycogen in the body will not greatly exceed 600 grams, and can well be as little as a quarter of that figure. When that amount is used up exhaustion sets in. Beyond this point, activity can proceed only at the low rate determined by mobilization and conversion of fat—corresponding to an oxygen supply of no more than a liter per minute, energy dissipation of around 300 calories an hour, and a speed of 3-4 m.p.h. In other words, any reasonably well-fed person can walk all day and every day without getting out of breath or feeling unduly tired. It is only when he speeds up that he runs into trouble. This is our concern here.

Two points stand out clearly:

1. Performance could be improved at distances below the mile by removing lactic acid.

2. Performance could be improved over the longer distances by increasing glycogen supply.

The best way to dispose of an acid is to neutralize it. Many attempts have been made to increase the maximum oxygen debt by feeding athletes alkaline materials before the race.

These experiments without exception have been failures for the following reasons: (1) the body has powerful controls built in to resist attempts to change its acid/alkaline balance; (2) it is almost certainly not lactic acid *as an acid* that causes trouble; and (3) it is no use neutralizing an athlete if he then feels too sick to run.

The maintenance and increase of glycogen, on the other hand, is both simple and effective. Glucose—often called *dextrose*—is a natural sugar. It is the form in which energy is transmitted inside the body. Carbohydrate foods are converted into glucose, which is carried in the blood to form glycogen in liver and muscle. Glycogen can be regarded as an insoluble form of glucose; the two are inconvertible and used interchangeably for energy production.

It would therefore seem obvious that the glycogen stock of the body could be conserved, and exhaustion warded off by eating glucose. This is in fact so. Dogs can run for 24 hours or more without apparent fatigue if given glucose every hour. Without glucose, they collapse exhausted—however well nourished—after a few hours.

Thus, before any athletic event, whether sprint or distance, care should be taken (1) to build up glycogen stores with a carbohydrate-rich diet for a few days before the event, and (2) where appropriate, to maintain those stores by eating glucose at appropriate intervals.

It may be asked: "Why, if all food is convertible into glucose, do you insist on glucose?" The great merit of it is that it is absorbed rapidly and directly into the bloodstream and is available for muscular use the moment it gets there. All other substances must undergo digestion, are absorbed more slowly, or must be converted into glucose after entering the bloodstream.

Glucose is the fastest-acting nutrient. Even so, one could wish it were faster still, for a snack of glucose takes about 30 minutes to produce its full effect. Its effect is shown by an increase in blood sugar of 50 percent or more. No harm will come from an occasional excess, for the kidneys automatically excrete into the bladder any amount more than twice the normal level.

Although the body controls the minimum blood sugar value until all glycogen is gone, there is much to be said for maintaining a higher level. In fact, the response of the body to exertion or stress is to mobilize glycogen and raise blood sugar. This is likely related to the fact that the effects of a slight deficiency in oxygen supply to the brain (as happens when the body goes into oxygen debt) are minimized by high blood sugar. This is again linked to the fact that there is a mental element in all fatigue, and that even purely mental fatigue is alleviated by glucose.

Therefore, although from the strictly energetic aspect no benefit is to be expected from eating glucose before events of less than two miles, there can be a real neurophysiological benefit even at the shortest distances. (Any effect in "single-effort" events will be purely psychological.) It must always be remembered that there will be a time lag of up to 30 minutes after eating. The amount needed is small—only a few grams (one or two tablets, if taken in tablet form).

For long distances, glucose is essential. It can be taken shortly before starting, and then perhaps every half-hour, according to personal taste and availability. The desirable amounts are fairly substantial. (Since it is less sweet than cane sugar, quite large amounts are easy to swallow.) Anything much less than an ounce is not likely to be worth the trouble. The choice as to whether the glucose should be taken in liquid or tablet form is up to the individual. Perhaps the most practical means of taking glucose is in on-the-run drinks.

Suppose now that a second event is to follow the next day. It is not possible to restore glycogen stores overnight—or even in two nights. And all athletes know what can result if one middle- or long-distance event follows another at too short an interval. The problem was, until very recently, insoluble in practical terms. But now a substance known as *fructose* has become available at a price that allows it to be eaten, and not just used for medicinal purposes.

Fructose—often called "fruit sugar" because it occurs commonly in fruit—looks just like glucose, but is about three times as sweet. Like glucose, fructose is absorbed rapidly and completely into the bloodstream when eaten. But, unlike glucose, there is no question of its being immediately available for muscular use. Its destiny is quite different than glucose. Fructose is rapidly and completely converted into glycogen. The speed of conversion is startling.

So the obvious way to build up glycogen stocks rapidly is to eat fructose. To replenish the body's stock of 1½ pounds of glycogen would require 1½ pounds of fructose—a lot of sugar to eat in an evening. But in fact glucose derived from the rest of the diet will play a substantial part in forming glycogen, as will body fat. So fructose should be taken for "topping off" glycogen stocks rather than as a major supply item. (Fructose also has the unusual property of increasing the speed at which glucose is converted into glycogen—thus providing a kind of bonus.)

How should fructose be taken? Any way you like, for it can replace ordinary sugar in nearly all foods. But, to keep things simple, fructose can be taken in beverages or on cereals—or perhaps best of all for sweetening fruit.

12
Blood Sugar Supplies

George Sheehan, M.D.

The fuel content of an ordinary 150-pound human being is approximately 166,200 calories—1,200 in carbohydrate, 25,000 in protein, and 140,000 in fat. Yet this 150-pounder, fortified by extra calories at breakfast, must have a coffee break two to three hours later or get the vapors.

Why? The answer is low blood sugar. Most of us suffer from it because we eat the wrong breakfast—or, if you go along with veteran marathoner Aldo Scandurra, from eating breakfast at all.

"When I get up the day of the Boston Marathon," Scandurra once told me, "I don't eat at all. I take a large glass of hot water, have a bowel movement, and I'm ready for that race at noon." And what about energy for that long 26 miles? "I have enough already stored up," he replied. "There's no sense upsetting my system with more."

Scandurra is physiologically correct. In the fasting person, the blood sugar stays in a straight line well within the normal range. Only after a meal does it rise, thereby calling for an outpouring of insulin (a hormone of energy storage). When the insulin accomplishes this task, the sugar level drops and you usually know it.

How? Well, you feel as if you need a coffee break. More specifically, that could range from fatigue and yawning or actual drowsiness on the one hand, to a feeling of jitteriness or a light sweat on the other. The treatment is usually coffee and a Danish. Other therapies include all those quick-energy foods and candies and drinks we see advertised in the press and on TV. The effect is almost immediate. Zing goes the blood sugar—back up and even past normal. This again calls on the insulin to deposit the extra calories. And thus we go on and on depositing high-octane fuel in an already full tank, depositing fat on top of fat, when all we had to do was call on the energy we already had stored for use.

Can this be done? Can low blood sugar be cured without diet or treated without jelly sandwiches, candy bars, and fruit juice? Can we raise our blood sugar any time we want to?

Why not? Children and athletes do. What do grammar-school students do at 10:30 in the morning when they get the same feeling that sends grown men and women to the kitchen or the snack bar? They have recess. They get out and raise a sweat, and in the process elevate their blood sugar. They then come back to the classroom renewed and intelligent, becoming more docile, more teachable. The transformation is a physiological one.

And what about the athlete? He has the same meal. He has been advised to have a relatively high carbohydrate meal before the event. If nothing else, it is more easily digested. Then he waits the two to three hours. Insulin, the hormone of energy storage, is doing its work. His blood sugar starts down. He begins to yawn (spectators mistakenly marvel at how casually he seems to be taking the race), or gets into a light, clammy perspiration. Does he then look around for food, something to raise his blood sugar? Of course not. He knows he is ready to release this power he has crammed into his muscles and liver. This is what these feelings mean to an athlete.

So he does the only appropriate thing, the natural thing for the human animal. He goes into physical action. That action, for reasons we did not know until recently, must be intense enough to cause sweating and prolonged enough to call on what has been described as that "miraculous refreshment and renewal of vigor"—the second wind.

We now read that there is a good scientific reason for all of this. The pancreas, which produces insulin, a hormone of energy storage, also produces *glucagon*, a hormone of energy release. Further, when the athlete exercises he stimulates the production of glucagon, with the result that all the fuel he has stashed away in the last meal—and the past week and past year, if necessary—begins to pour out into the blood. *Voila,* the blood sugar rises.

There is a time, the Bible says, for everything. There is a time for low blood sugar. There is time for high blood sugar. There is a time for insulin. There is a time for glucagon. There is a time for meat, a time for bread, and a time for nothing at all. The problem is finding the right time.

13
On Foods and Fasting

Athletes as a group subscribe wholeheartedly to the "you-are-what-you-eat" school of thinking. Reasoning runs like this: Exercise burns up calories. Therefore, the exercising athlete must eat more than the average person so he'll have more calories available for energy. And since muscles are doing the work, plenty of muscle-food (meat protein) is needed to keep them working.

This sounds logical enough. Three square meals every day, heavy on calories and meats, represents the conventional means of feeding athletes. But scientific evidence to the contrary is mounting. In several significant ways, the studies are indicating that the athlete is what he *doesn't* eat.

Skipping meals (fasting) and skipping meats (vegetarianism) are still generally regarded as food fads, with no place in athletic diet. Not eating certain "essential" foods, or not eating at all, for extended periods are self-defeating according to some so-called authorities. At best, these practices have no measurable effect on athletic performance say others.

However, a number of diet-endurance tests performed in Europe indicate otherwise. The conclusions have practical value to runners—particularly distance runners. Swiss doctor Ralph Bircher reviewed three studies on fasting and protein consumption for the German magazine *Leichtathletik.* The research isn't new. Two of the experiments are 30 years old, and the other occurred nearly a decade ago. But until recently they were buried in technical journals and were lost to most of the people who needed this information.

The first test deals with fasting. In 1964, a group of 19 Swedes took a walk from Kalmar to Stockholm—a distance of over 300 miles, which they covered at the rate of 30 miles a day. Most of the men, aged 18 to 53, were sedentary workers. They had no background as endurance athletes. They ate no food at all during the 10-day walk.

"Insane, foolish, impossible, we are inclined to say," Bircher notes, "because we live for the most part in the belief that our daily need for food must be constantly stilled—even when one is doing nothing, not to mention during such a long walk. We are convinced that otherwise we would soon fold up."

Though their average weight loss was about 15 pounds, all the walkers completed the test. "The happy, natural appearance and obvious liveliness of the walkers at the finish, and a minute examination both showed that they were all in the best of health."

In this case, the walkers proved one of Ernst van Aaken's contentions: that the body is perfectly capable of "living off its own resources" for extended periods, and in fact even thrives on it.

The second test involves a sudden shift from cooked and processed foods to raw, fresh ones. This was done back in 1933, with three young sports students as subjects. The test lasted six weeks. During the first two weeks, the athletes ate their normal mixed diet (which included approximately 100 grams of protein, 150 grams of fat, 230 grams of carbohydrate, and 14½ grams of salt daily). They trained to the point of best performance. Then they made an abrupt shift in diet. They changed to raw foods (fruits, vegetables, nuts—with very small amounts of milk and eggs). Protein consumption was cut in half, and salt intake by almost 90 percent.

Following the shift to this unfamiliar diet, there were more tests (rowing, diving, long-distance running, gymnastics). "The results surpassed all expectations," Bircher says. "In the three weeks of pure fresh foods, there was no decrease whatsoever in athletic performances. Metabolism was in continuous balance, no digestive difficulties at all, increased sensation of well-being. We see that demanding physical performance can continue unreduced even after sudden—almost grotesque—inversion of the diet. We also see that with minimal protein (50 grams), best performances can still be possible."

The third test centers on protein consumption. Does the working runner need more than normal amounts to keep his muscles operating effectively? Another 1933 study indicates just the opposite. Heavy protein intake may in fact *impede* performance.

For one thing, Bircher says, "the caloric need grows by one-fourth when one adds protein to the extent customary in sports." This is apparently because more energy is required to assimilate protein than to break down other food substances. One of the protein researchers who made this discovery was a mountain climber. In one high-mountain experiment, he limited his protein consumption to whole wheat (7-8 percent protein)—and ate no cheese, eggs, or meat.

Bircher says, "In this way, the large, heavy man's caloric intake dropped from 3000-3600 per day to 2400, and thirst and perspiration largely disappeared. His muscular performance increased by 20-30% as tested, and the need for oxygen sank by 10%, which at great altitudes naturally proved quite useful. Performance was optimal, and above all an extraordinary increase in endurance and recovery ability appeared. The rest days, previously unavoidable after days-long strenuous high altitude effort, could be omitted, as a night's rest sufficed and shorter pauses were able to replace longer rest periods."

Lower total calories means lower weight—usually a positive factor for runners. If a runner can lose weight and at the same time increase energy, oxygen intake, recovery rate, and well-being (these tests strongly indicate one can), certain foods are worth skipping.

14
Eating on Yoga Terms

George Beinhorn

I started running in 1969, two years after becoming a vegetarian. This makes it hard for me to say what effect a vegetarian diet has had on my running. I do, however, have the strong feeling that natural foods are the most efficient way to get the right nutrients to the cells, and that a pure-foods diet keeps the organs of assimilation, crystallization, and elimination in the best health. But one thing at a time, and from the beginning.

It takes great interest to change your diet. You eat the same things for X number of years, and are bound by very strong habits. No one can talk you into being a vegetarian or fruitarian, or not eating white flour, etc. It takes a keen personal sense of the reasons why this is the best thing to do. Why, indeed, do we make any changes in our lives? Because we expect, rightly or not, that they will make us happier or healthier. Well, this is why I began to change my diet.

I was miserable, emotionally drained by chaotic human relationships; physically a mess from two major surgeries and irrational, destructive habits; mentally stale and tired from too much booking and a crash effort to finish my master's thesis. After graduation and an extended rest period, I began to do research again, on the most efficient and surefire means of having a deeply meaningful, if not overtly happy life. This led me, inevitably, to yoga, a system of physical, mental, and spiritual culture that has been tested for over 5,000 years. In yoga, all systems are interrelated; the physical side has its mental and spiritual effects.

The yoga diet is simplicity itself. That is why it is rather difficult to follow, as we are not often used to reducing our behavior to simplicity. The *Bhagavad-Gita* says that there are three qualities universally present in various mixtures everywhere in this world: (1) the negative or destructive, (2) the activating, and (3) the soothing or spiritual. Foods can be classified according to these qualities:

1. In rotten foods, such as stinky cheeses and thousand-year-old eggs, or even stale vegetables, we easily see the negative, degenerative quality. The yogis say that these foods tend to create certain corresponding qualities of the mind: a lazy, sullen, sadistic, destructive disposition. Let me qualify that right now: the effect of food is by no means to override and dominate well-developed personal qualities. We all know wonderfully cheerful, positive people who eat *tamasic* foods, as they are called. This class of food also extends to many of the items currently under fire by "inner ecologists," such as white flour, over-cooked vegetables, and meats.

2. The stimulating, or *rajasic*, category includes foods that taste sharp, acid, bitter, or sour. These are said to produce a nervous, jumpy mind and disposition. One example is salt, which is known to cause hypertension and acts as a thyroid stimulant. Try to give up salt. You'll find out that it is a strongly addictive stimulant. Others are hot peppers, vinegar, and mustard. Again, avoiding these foods won't make you calm and peaceful; nor will eating them necessarily make you jumpy and irritable if you have an inclination toward calmness. The *Bhagavad-Gita* only gives this advice for those who want to put their body systems in a state that will not interfere with the cultivation of mental states that are conducive to happiness.

3. The third, spiritual, or *sattwic*, type of food is easily identified. These are the foods that appeal most to our senses of smell, sight, and taste, discounting the unnatural appeal to stimulation and gluttony of the other two categories: fruit, fresh vegetables, nuts, and grains. Think of a hamburger with plenty of mustard and relish, then a bowl of fresh, sliced peaches with honey, or blueberries, or watermelon. Which seems more soothing, pleasing to the eye, easily digested?

There are two additional tests that tell what kind of food is most natural for man: (1) the ratio of the length of the intestinal tract to the distance between the mouth and the anus, and (2) the tooth structure. Without elaborating, these are specific to each animal, including human beings, according to the kind of food on which the animal thrives. The teeth, of course, have to be a certain shape in order to chew and tear the characteristic food. And the intestinal tract must not be too long, or the food will begin to rot before it leaves the animal's body, becoming a festering ground for disease bacteria. By these tests, man is a fruit-and-nut eater.

To return to my own case, after struggling with the initial change I began to feel much more energy. My body felt "magnetized." There isn't a better word. I got tired much less frequently. When I did start running I had no problems related to nutrition. It was a struggle to work up to easy three-mile runs, as it is for everyone. But I never felt a lack of energy that kept me from recovering from one day to the next, working eight hours as usual, and gradually lengthening my runs.

My specific diet is as follows. I don't find it monotonous at all, because I have by five-year habit returned to natural tastes in food. Things that a meat-and-spice-eating person wouldn't look twice at are delicious to me. Oranges, for instance, and most other fruits are the most delicious dessert items I can imagine.

Breakfast: (heaviest meal of the day) two handfuls of nuts; four or five large tablespoons of sesame seed mixed with wheat germ and honey; six to eight dates or prunes (unsulphured); an orange; maybe a lemon or some pineapple.

Lunch: a handful of a different kind of nuts than were eaten at breakfast; pineapple if I hadn't eaten any at breakfast; fruit juice (usually grapefruit or apple); another orange.

After-work snack: a pint to a quart of raw skim milk; fruit; maybe an orange; a small glass of apple juice or more if it's hot; a carrot or two.

Dinner: A big salad made of a base of romaine lettuce and raw spinach leaves, plus whatever else my creative impulses decide (alfalfa sprouts, tomato, etc.); I use a homemade dressing of soy oil, garlic, herbs, and vinegar (the vinegar will soon be switched to lemon juice, as I think it's hard on the kidneys).

I don't want anyone else to follow this diet. I doubt that anyone would. The point I will make is that I get along on this, with no meat and potatoes, and run with good energy. I run 8 to 10 miles four days a week, take two easy days of 2-3 miles, and go out in the hills for a run of 17-22 miles on a Saturday or Sunday. I intend to use the van Aaken run-walk system to learn to go more than 25 miles on a weekend run, as I think that most of the trouble at 20 miles is due to the body's never having been forced to learn to switch over to conversion of stored fats after it runs out of glycogen. I vary the basic diet radically after a long run, especially on a hot day. Then there is no question about heading for the nearest store to get some fruit. I've found berries to be the most refreshing postrun food, especially strawberries and blueberries. Raw milk also seems to be a good recovery drink. I have no scientific evidence of this, just personal experience repeated many times.

Ideally, I fast one day a week, and three days once a month. Recently I have begun fasting until noon with good results. I believe fasting is necessary to clean out the body from time to time. During a fast I drink a lot of orange juice, and take a herbal laxative. The effects are predominantly mental for me, but there are good effects on my running. I feel more energy during the first run while fasting. The digestive organs do a lot of work to push food through 30 feet of tubing, and I think when I stop eating this energy is freed for running. I've also fasted on the day of a race, getting my best time for five miles. My longest fast while continuing to run was four days, and the last run was a real flop. I see no need to keep on training through a long fast except as an experiment, never pushing it beyond what feels tolerable in order to preserve energy for the body's inner cleansing work.

For about three months I loaded up on vitamin E pills, magnesium, and potassium. I noticed no change at all, and therefore guess I am getting enough of these in the nuts I eat.

One serious mistake I made as a vegetarian was in not getting enough of the right kind of protein. I cut out milk completely, as well as wheat and any soybean products. I don't want to generalize my experience, as I have read about contradictory experiences, but after a year and a half without milk, etc., I began to have poor concentration and a kind of lightheadedness, which I was told were symptoms of protein deficiency. Sure enough, when I started getting more milk I recovered within about three weeks. I now get along very well on about 70 grams of protein a day, but I'm careful to include two or more foods in my daily diet that give me at least the basic 10 amino acids—from which the body is able to manufacture the rest.

Since I've been a vegetarian trying to control food intake, my weight has not varied more than five pounds up or down.

The high-carbohydrate race preparation formula has produced good results for me on one occasion, and wretched runs on two others. I believe that in the two unhappy cases I overdid it, eating so much carbohydrate food that my heartbeat and breathing rates increased, making sleep shallow and unrestful, and sapping the energy I would have used to race. My experiences have convinced me there must be moderation, even in this kind of radical diet.

Part III
The Body's Regulators

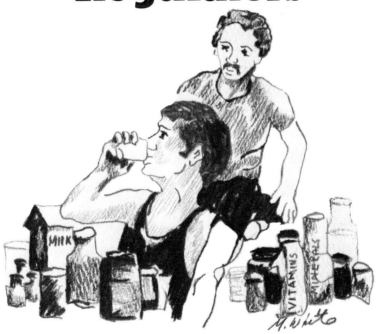

15
Let's Drink to That

Immediately before, during, and after running, the runner's drinking habits should concern him more than what he eats. Calories only burn up at the rate of about 100 per mile in a distance run; this means it takes 35 miles to lose a pound of flesh. On the other hand, a pound of fluid may drain away in as little as two miles; on hot days, the pace may be faster yet.

David Costill is perhaps the leading American exercise physiologist studying runners. Dr. Costill has tested fluid losses in distance men, both in his laboratory at Ball State University and in actual races. Costill says, "When a man loses 2% or more of his body weight by sweating, his ability to perform prolonged exhaustive exercise is drastically impaired. During our laboratory test, we recorded weight losses of nearly 7% of the runner's body weight."

Fluid loss (we use the word *fluid* here because it isn't simply pure water that the runner is losing; the water contains many dissolved minerals) hits athletes two ways:

1. *They get thirsty, obviously.* This indicates that the liquid supply is running low and needs to be replaced. If thirst isn't at least partially quenched, performance will suffer.
2. *Internal temperatures rise.* When temperatures get too high, performance suffers this way, too. In extreme cases, heat exhaustion or heat stroke can result.

Costill found in his testing that thirst isn't an accurate guide to fluid needs. He also discovered that a runner can't possibly fill his needs while the run or race is on.

In a *Distance Running News* article, Costill wrote, "At the 1968 US Olympic marathon trial, we recorded weight losses as large as 13.5 pounds. The average weight loss of the top 10 finishers was 9.3 pounds. We were amazed at the small amount of fluid drunk in the course of 2½ to three hours of running. The average volume of fluid taken at each of the feeding stations was 1.5 ounces. That means that these men were only replacing about 0.5 of the 9.3 pounds that they were losing."

The runners, he says, were only drinking enough to quiet their immediate thirst. This doesn't come close to matching the body's true demand. Costill says, too, that the placement of drinking stations in long-distance races is a problem. According to the physiologist, by the time a man gets his first drink, he may already have lost more than three pounds. In the laboratory, the subjects took 3.5 ounces every five minutes during their runs—and came through their runs with less weight loss and fewer dehydration symptoms.

Acute dehydration, occurring during a run, hurts performance in that run. However, losses are usually repaid soon afterward. Costill's bigger concern is with *chronic dehydration.*

"Large body water losses incurred on consecutive days may cause an accumulated weight and fluid loss," he says. "Man generally relies on his thirst to control body fluid balance. Unfortunately, this mechanism is far from accurate. In laboratory tests that required about eight pounds of sweat loss, we found that thirst was temporarily satisfied by as little as one pound of water. Total replacement of body weight may take several days unless the runner forces himself to drink more than is desired.

"Chronic dehydration can drastically damage a runner's endurance capacity by lowering his tolerance to fatigue, reducing his ability to sweat, elevating his rectal temperature and increasing the stress on his circulatory system."

Costill mentions here that a daily weight check is a better indicator of dehydration than is thirst. "If you note a two- or three-pound decrease in body weight from morning to morning, efforts should be made to increase your fluid intake. You need not worry about drinking too much fluid, because your kidneys will unload the excess water in a matter of a few hours."

Another of Costill's tests determined: (1) the amount of

fluid absorbed by the body during exercise, and (2) the effect of liquid intake on internal temperatures. Four test subjects—all national class middle- and long-distance runners—went through a series of three treadmill runs. They went the equivalent of six-minute mile pace, meaning that each run was a hard 20-miler. During each test run, the athletes gulped 4.5 pounds of water or Gatorade (which contains sodium chloride, potassium, phosphorus, and glucose).* They drank at five-minute intervals for most of each run. "To add to the pain of the situation," Costill says, "the runners' stomachs were aspirated [pumped] immediately after each test to determine how much fluid remained in the stomach."

He found that "only about 81% of the 0.54 gallons ingested had actually been absorbed from the stomach. We have estimated that a runner will lose about 3.7 pounds per hour, but he can only remove about 1.8 pounds of water from his stomach in the same period. That means that regardless of how much a runner drinks, it will be impossible for him to keep up with the weight being lost by sweating."

Still, the conclusion was that during a run such as this—a simulated 20 mile run—drinking fluids will "significantly benefit" a runner. That's because it lowers the internal temperatures. Costill says, "Rectal temperatures were two degrees (F) lower when the runners drank fluids than when they did not. Amby Burfoot's internal temperature reached 105.5 degrees when he ran without fluids, but leveled off at 103.6 degrees when he drank either of the two fluids (water or Gatorade). Since a body temperature above 104.5 can cause extreme distress and possible collapse, this cooling quality of ingested fluids could be of paramount value on a warm day."

Summarizing Costill's findings:

1. He strongly recommends drinking during long runs and races—as much to reduce body heat as to ward off thirst.

2. He would do away with restrictions on distance-race drinking stations, letting runners take in all they want.

3. After and between hard runs, he thinks the best way to

---

* Other electrolyte solutions, such as Body Punch and ERG, are preferred by most runners.

avoid dehydration is to watch one's weight; sudden losses mean trouble, and corrective action should be taken.

4. Costill adds that fluids are retained or replaced more effectively with electrolyte solutions (such as Gatorade) than with plain water.

16
Do Runners Need Salt?

Common table salt—sodium chloride, in chemical terminology—is the subject of controversy. Does it help or hurt running performances? Conventional wisdom goes like this: sweat is salty, so heavily sweating individuals need extra salt to replace what is lost; if they don't get it, they risk fatigue symptoms, muscle cramping, and even heat exhaustion or stroke.

In the previous article, Dr. David Costill said, "Attempts should be made to drink fluids that will be retained by the body. After acute dehydration, drinking water will only produce a partial rehydration. The ingredient needed to improve the retention of water is sodium chloride."

There isn't total agreement in the scientific community on this claim. Other researchers are saying that salt isn't the complete answer—and, in fact, that it may not be as essential a supplement to the athlete's diet as was once believed.

Dr. Kenneth Cooper, originator and popularizer of the "aerobics" program, tested three-quarters of a million volunteers while doing his research. His is the largest single body of data on running physiology. Several of his tests have centered on the loss and replacement of fluid electrolytes—which include not only sodium chloride, but also potassium, calcium, and magnesium. Cooper has tentatively concluded that sodium chloride may be the least important of the four, and that magnesium is most critical. His test of marathoners showed no significant sodium chloride loss during races, but a heavy drain on magnesium supplies. Cooper conducted much of his research in the hot and steamy Texas summer. One could reasonably expect runners to need extra salt under these conditions—perhaps in the form of salt tablets. Cooper says no.

One of the greatest factors leading to heat stress problems is inadequate fluid replacement, particularly in a heat acclimatized subject. Salt tablets alone may do more harm than good if taken without adequate fluids. As a means of preventing heat stress, I always encourage adequate fluid replacement *first* and salt intake *second*.

Most runners can compensate for the salt loss, once they are heat acclimatized, by merely adding extra salt to their food. In fact, most of our noon runners in San Antonio did not find it necessary to take salt tablets, even though three- to five-mile runs were quite common in high temperature, high humidity conditions so prevalent during the summer. On no occasion did one of our runners suffer a heat stress syndrome.

Two other American researchers did their studies in hot weather areas, where salt intake should have been most important. Physicians James Schamadan and W. D. Snively tested teenagers working in the scorching fields of Israel and Arizona. Temperatures frequently were about 100 degrees. Schamadan's and Snively's subjects, who were doing longer but less intense work than found in running, developed serious potassium deficits even though they were eating adequately and were getting supplementary salt. The potassium deficiency disappeared when they switched to high-potassium foods and stopped taking salt tablets.

The two doctors concluded that high salt intake accelerates sweating, and in the process "washes out" other essential electrolytes besides salt. They say some of the confusion about high salt intake may have developed because the substance "probably relieves heat exhaustion at the onset, but then as the body's potassium reserves drop it [salt] exerts the opposite effect."

Dr. George Sheehan says one effect of adapting to heat is that the salt content of the sweat drops almost to insignificance. He claims that at best the extra salt may be wasted, noting, "The body quickly throws off excess." This "throwing off" process, in turn, could contribute to the situation Schamadan and Snively were talking about. Dr. Sheehan, a world-record veteran distance runner himself, says, "I have been on a low-salt, high potassium diet for years, and have been satisfied with my performances. How I would do on salt I'm not sure, and frankly I'm not about to try."

17
Victories Over Heat

In 1965, Tom Osler went off the salt shaker. He was then, he admits, "a terrible hot day runner." But he decided that salt deficiency wasn't the reason. He says he finished his runs looking like a pillar of salt, having it caked on his face, neck, arms, and shoes. Tom's experience told him his diet was too high in salt. He read a physiology textbook and it concurred. It said the average American diet is "unnaturally high" in salt, and that the body's needs can be met from natural sources—without turning to the salt shaker.

Osler figured he had an unnecessary addiction, so he stopped. There were immediate results.

- Body weight dropped several pounds.
- He worked more efficiently in heat.
- He sweated less, and the sweat was less salty.

The real test of his low-salt diet ("low by American standards; natural by God's standard") came two years later. Tom ran the National AAU marathon championship, which incorporated the Pan-American Games Trial. The race came to be known as the "Holyoke Massacre" because so many runners fell to the 97-degree noonday heat and humidity near 100 percent. It was so hot, he says, that his shoes made a clicking sound as they stuck to the melting asphalt. Osler finished fourth in that race, while most of the big names dropped out. He said this convinced him that he'd gone from one of the worst hot weather runners to one of the best, simply by cutting out table salt.

"After the race," Osler says, "I took my friend Ted Corbitt aside and with great eagerness announced my amazing discovery. Ted, in his usual quiet, reserved manner, grinned and told me that he had known this for many years—and had himself been an advocate of low salt diets."

Corbitt is the U.S. record holder at 50 and 100 miles, both set when he was past 40 years old. Not coincidentally, Ted is known as one of the country's most effective hot weather runners.

Fred Grace's salt-free experience goes back even further. Grace is the holder of many world age-group records for runners over 70. He claims he hasn't had so much as a headache since he was 13, and he attributes this to his combined exercise-diet program.

"I haven't used salt for over 30 years," Grace says. "Why haven't I died? Because everything we eat and drink contains salt. And added salt causes strokes."

Osler warns, however, that suddenly eliminating excess salt can temporarily cause trouble. The body has become dependent on these large does and has to be weaned away carefully. He says men working in extreme heat may initially experience muscle cramps, dizziness, and nausea. According to Osler, the best time to cut down on salt is during the cool weather months. Then, when summer comes again, the runner will be adjusted. He'll surprise himself at how well he copes with heat and humidity.

18

Drinks for the Road

Peter Van Handel

Numerous articles have discussed the importance of stored carbohydrate (glycogen) for endurance running, and have presented protocols that runners may follow in an attempt to "carbohydrate-pack." It has also been emphasized that this technique does not benefit everyone and, indeed, may not be advisable for certain individuals.

As would be expected, there is a large group of runners who, for various reasons, cannot or do not wish to "pack." However, based on the available experimental and practical evidence, we have to concede that *all* runners need to maintain adequate carbohydrate levels during endurance exercise. This article is directed at these athletes—the ones who are asking themselves, "How do I insure that adequate carbohydrate is available to the muscles if I can't carbohydrate-pack?"

The answer is obvious. You take sugar or some other form of carbohydrate while "on the road." Hundreds of runners answer the gun with dextrose tablets tucked away someplace in their uniforms. The most common form of carbohydrate ingestion occurs in the form of a cup of Gatorade, ERG, or some other drink every few miles. However, there are problems with taking carbohydrates on the run, and for all practical purposes these cannot be separated from the problems associated with fluid intake. Therefore, this discussion centers on the drinking of carbohydrate solutions.

Basically, most runners drink the various commercially available "ades" or other homemade solutions to provide quick energy. I've seen national caliber endurance athletes take honey on a spoon in an attempt to delay fatigue during a long race. Others drink both for the energy supplies and to help delay or prevent dehydration and the symptoms of heat stress when the runs are held in hot weather.

But a nagging question remains: "Does the substance you are taking during the run to provide energy really do the job?" Unfortunately, there is not a simple "yes" or "no" answer since there are several complicating factors.

Generally speaking, the following are true: (1) the greater the volume of fluid in the stomach, the faster it tends to leave the stomach, but (2) the more sugar or carbohydrate the fluid has, the longer it takes to leave the stomach, and (3) these factors interact in an athlete drinking carbohydrate solutions during a race. The importance of this is that if the fluid is in your stomach, the carbohydrate present can't get to your muscles.

Let's examine these factors in greater detail.

Effects of volume of fluid in the stomach. The falling off of pace and the fatigue felt as the carbohydrate stores become depleted isn't due to a sudden drop in energy supplies. Rather, evidence indicates a gradual and continuous depletion of carbohydrate stores. At the same time, large sweat losses may occur. This, combined with carbohydrate depletion, and the problems of "voluntary dehydration," usually means that by the time fluid is available to the athlete, it is too late to solve the immediate problems. The dehydration and fatigue have already started to set in. Drinking a large volume of fluid loaded with "energy" can't bring the body back to a normal state, since it takes a relatively long time for the material to leave the stomach.

Indeed, Dr. David Costill has reported that national-class runners attempting to consume large volumes of a sugar solution during runs at competitive pace complained of stomach discomfort (fullness) and an inability to consume fluids after the first few feedings. This was in spite of the fluid need as evidenced by subjective reports of muscle and nervous system fatigue, and by the sweat losses.

While volume is the least important of the three factors mentioned, it does have some effects on performance, especially when combined with the other two factors. Therefore, based on our experience with distance runners, we suggest that drinking approximately one pint 10 minutes *before* the run, and then supplementing with frequent drinks (every 10-15 minutes) of small volume, is the best procedure to follow.

Effects of sugar concentration. The next question is, "What do we drink?" I've already mentioned that in general the more carbohydrate in the drink, the longer it takes the solution to get out of the stomach. The energy available in the drink cannot be used until the carbohydrate leaves the stomach and enters the blood from the small intestine. Numerous studies have shown that salt solutions leave the stomach very rapidly, and the addition of even small amounts of sugar can drastically slow down the rate of emptying. This delays the movement of water into the blood.

During endurance running in the heat, prevention of dehydration and heat stress is of utmost importance. Carbohydrate supplementation is secondary. Therefore, under these conditions the sugar content of the drink should be minimal, so that water can rapidly enter the circulating blood.

Various commercially available drinks claim to have everything you need to take during an endurance run. Unfortunately, there is little hard data to back up these claims. In fact, the evidence seems to indicate that champion distance runners are able to complete a marathon with little or no fluid intake. However, in the process they sustain water losses of 6-10 percent of their body weight and rectal temperatures in excess of 105 degrees (F). This obviously places severe demands on the runner and exposes him to the hazards of muscle cramps, heat exhaustion, and heat stroke.

Research studies do not agree on the effects of carbohydrate solutions on the body's energy-producing mechanisms during endurance events. Costill reports that the carbohydrate taken during severe endurance exercise does not reach the muscles in significant amounts. The little that is used to produce energy takes 20-30 minutes to reach the muscles after it enters the stomach. This tends to support the idea of drinking *before* the run and then supplementing at frequent intervals.

Costill's data also indicates that while the contribution of the ingested carbohydrate to muscle metabolism is minimal, it does seem to conserve the liver carbohydrate stores by maintaining blood sugar. The blood sugar and liver stores are seemingly used to prevent brain and nervous system fatigue.

While Costill's data points to insignificant use of carbohydrate by the muscles, another research study estimated that 60-80 percent of the carbohydrate used after the feeding came from the drink. Here again, though, the time from intake until utilization was rather long. Factors such as intensity and type of work play a role in these studies, so comparisons between the two are difficult.

Other supportive evidence for preevent fluid intake comes from the 1968 Olympic 50-kilometer cross-country ski champion, who was reported to have drunk more than a quart of 40 percent sugar water before the start of his race. This seems to indicate a wide variability in the tolerance to drinking carbohydrate solutions, as most people could not swallow a 40 percent sugar solution (commercially available drinks are about 5-10 percent carbohydrate).

There seems to be no reason for eating dextrose tablets, honey, etc., as fatigue sets in during a race. The material remains in the stomach too long to be of any practical value in supplying immediate energy. The benefits of dextrose would be felt some 30 minutes after consumption, and it also tends to keep water in the stomach.

Effects of exercise severity. Research has shown that exercise tasks exceeding approximately 70 percent of the individual's maximal ability to use oxygen inhibit emptying of the stomach. Champion distance men can run an entire marathon in excess of 80 percent of this capacity. For example, in tests on Derek Clayton in our laboratory it was shown that the pace for his 2:08 marathon was in excess of 86 percent of his maximal ability.

Obviously, not all of us can function at this level. The point is that many runners can exceed the level where stomach emptying becomes affected by the work intensity. The carbohydrate (and water) tends to stay in the stomach longer.

Let's tie things together at this point. I've already stated that the factors of volume of fluid in the stomach, the sugar content of the fluid, and the severity of exercise all interact in the athlete who drinks on the run. This interaction is more complex than I've made it seem, so research data on the topic of fluid intake during exercise is hard to evaluate. In turn, no specific recommendations can be made at this time concerning how much, when, and what a runner needs to provide energy and prevent dehydration during a long run.

However, based on the evidence to date and our own experience with distance runners, we can make the following suggestions:

1. In order to minimize dehydration, a pint of fluid should be consumed 10 minutes *before* competition.
2. In order to prevent stomach distress (fullness), and to promote maximal entry of the fluid into the blood, the drink should contain very little carbohydrate (less than 2.5 percent). This amount is adequate for energy production and use by the nervous system.
3. The fluid should be taken at 10- to 15-minute intervals during the run in amounts of about one-half pint.
4. Scheduling of races should be such that they are held during the cool hours of the day to minimize heat stress problems. The present situation seems to benefit the officials, sponsors, and spectators, and is not in the best interests of the athlete.

References

Costill, D. L. "Health Hazards During Distance Running." *American College Sports Medicine News* 8 (1973):6.

Costill, D. L. "Water and Electrolytes." *Ergogenic Aids and Muscular Performance.* New York: Academic Press, 1972, pp. 293-319.

Costill, D. L.; Bennett, A.; Branam, G.; and Eddy, P. "Glucose Ingestion at Rest and During Prolonged Exercise." *Journal of Applied Physiology* 34 (1973):764-69.

Costill, D. L.; Kammer, W.; and Fisher, A. "Fluid Ingestion During Distance Running." *Archives of Environmental Health* 21 (1970):520-25.

Costill, D. L., and Sparks, K. "Rapid Fluid Replacement Following Thermal Dehydration." *Journal of Applied Physiology* 34 (1973):299-303.

Davenport, H. W. *Physiology of the Digestive Tract.* Chicago: Year Book Medical Publishers, Inc., 1961.

19
Drinking Legislation

*"A competitor taking refreshments at a place other than the refreshments points appointed by the organizers renders himself liable to disqualification."**

That was the rule in long-distance races. It was generally ignored in all but the biggest national and international competitions, but was still the rule. Officials at all races have the power to enforce it, whether or not they use it.

This is what it said in the International Amateur Athletic Federation handbook—rule 165, section five: "Refreshments shall be provided by organizers of the race at approximately 11 kilometers or seven miles, and thereafter at approximately every five kilometers or three miles." The rule further states that "no refreshment may be carried or taken by a competitor other than that provided or approved by the organizers."

The runner was put in the position of (1) suffering because of an apparently arbitrary rule, or (2) breaking the rule for the sake of his performance and health. This is particularly true on warm days.

David Costill's tests indicated that neither subjective feelings of thirst nor the international rule took into account the body's true fluid needs. He says that by the time the runner felt thirsty and could drink, it may have been too late to do much good. According to Costill, "We have been led to conclude that international rules and the feeding habits during marathon races make the practice of drinking fluids totally ineffective. That is to say that the current methods of taking fluids during a marathon race do little more than satisfy the runner's thirst temporarily."

* This rule was finally changed by the International Amateur Athletic Federation for the 1976 Olympics. Until that time, this was the rule in long-distance races.

Costill's test subjects had the most success when they drank 3½ ounces of liquid every five minutes of their runs—starting in the first five minutes and continuing to drink until the last half-hour. "While this technique appears to be the most ideal method for replacing fluids during a race," he says, "current international marathon rules prohibit feedings before 11 kilometers. It is therefore possible that by the time a runner is able to begin replacing his fluid losses, he may have already lost more than three pounds."

Running drinks help to replace water, electrolytes, and energy. These things don't happen immediately. There is a certain time lag while the body processes the fluids. Experts on the subject say it takes 30 minutes or more to get the full effect from a water-mineral-glucose drink. This fact means that for runners:

1. The drinks do little or no physiological good in races shorter than six miles, even if they're taken in the first minute of the run.
2. If you follow the rules and take the first drink at seven miles, you don't get full benefit from it until you've gone perhaps 12 miles. By then, as Costill says, you're already in severe fluid debt.

One way to get around both of these things and be well watered in short races or the early miles of long ones is to drink *before* the run. Remember the half-hour time lag, and plan the drink for maximum good later on. Bill Gookin, the inventor of "Gookinaid" or ERG, follows this practice in his own races. Even before the shortest races, he drinks a half-cup of his product "to take the dryness out of my mouth." He reports nothing but good effects.

Dr. George Sheehan adds a warning: "Pre-race drinks (sodium chloride-potassium-sugar mixture) may be helpful. But the body quickly throws off excess, so don't rely on this completely."

The best solution was to change the drinking rule, which apparently had no scientific basis. Long-distance bicyclists carry their own drinks as they ride, and swig from their bottles whenever they want. This isn't practical for runners, but the idea is sound. Drinks should be available when runners need them—before they think they need them—and these needs don't follow any pattern that can be set down in a rule book.

20
The Magnesium Drain

It wasn't the most inviting prospect before and after a hard marathon. Dr. Kenneth Cooper, the developer and popularizer of the "aerobics" program, asked for blood donors. He wanted to see what happened in the runner's blood during a marathon. Surprisingly he got the necessary number of volunteers, and the test produced potentially valuable results.

Cooper did his testing at the 1969 Boston Marathon. His eight volunteers all gave samples of their blood an hour before the start. Then they ran. The temperature during the race was mild (55-60 degrees), so heat didn't create unusual havoc with the runners' fluid levels. They drank less than a pint of liquid apiece while running, so liquid replacement was minimal.

As soon as they finished—and before they ate or drank—Cooper sampled their blood again. He checked for mineral changes in the blood serum. Sodium, potassium, calcium, and magnesium were the electrolytes in which he was most interested.

Running drinks contain combinations of the first three—sodium, potassium, and calcium—but until recently magnesium hasn't gotten much attention. Cooper's findings, however, indicate that magnesium should find a more important place for itself in the food and drink of long-distance runners. He doesn't make any wild claims for the substance, but spells its role in cautious, scientific language. (Two running drinks, Body Punch and ERG, contain compounds of magnesium.)

"The data [from the test at Boston] show that all subjects exhibited a significant *rise* in serum sodium and potassium immediately after the marathon run. No significant change was noted in either serum chloride or serum calcium. There was a significant *fall* in serum magnesium after the run."

Cooper noted that it is unusual for potassium levels to rise while magnesium levels drop, since the activities of the two usually run parallel. He hinted that potassium may be rushing into the bloodstream from cellular storage to overcompensate for the increased demand. It isn't made clear why the same thing doesn't happen with magnesium. Perhaps, he says, it is because the cells release potassium easier than magnesium, or magnesium flushes out of the system faster.

In any event, magnesium losses through sweating are quite high. Cooper says, "Sweating could possibly account for considerable loss of total body magnesium. It is of interest to note that after the marathon run some of the participants complained of nausea and muscle cramps. These symptoms may in part be due to the magnesium changes noted."

Cooper concludes: "In sweating, many electrolytes are lost from the body. Replacement solutions of various types have been advocated for athletic participants, but to our knowledge most of these solutions do not contain significant quantities of magnesium. From this study it would appear that magnesium is perhaps depleted to a greater extent after a marathon run than some of the other electrolytes, and that replacement solutions containing magnesium as well as other electrolyes, should be evaluated to replace this deficit."

Cooper says he has talked with marathoners who supplement their diet with a commercial product called Dolomite, which contains calcium and magnesium. Another possibility, suggested by physician-marathoner J. Karr Taylor, is Magnesium Plus. In natural form, magnesium is available from a number of food sources. (See accompanying chart.)

One big problem with magnesium is that it passes through the body easily. Magnesium is lost through the feces, perhaps more than through sweat. When the mineral is taken in high doses, it tends to promote diarrhea. So the runner under stress taking extra magnesium and (already prone to diarrhea) may lose in two ways.

Dr. Taylor did an informal test with distance runners. "Each runner ran at varying distances and saved stool for a week at each distance," he says. "In almost every case, there was a rather remarkable step-wise increase in the loss of magnesium via the stool—not the sweat. It seems at least possible that the stool is the major avenue of magnesium loss in long distance runners, and the actual presence of intraluminal magnesium may well explain the observed absence of constipative difficulties in distance runners."

Taylor adds that daily fecal losses of magnesium average 138 milligrams, but "in the distance runner this loss may increase by from 50 to 100%." He says Magnesium Plus seems to produce less diarrhea than Dolomite, and that magnesium taken in natural-foods form has less effect yet.

Long before the magnesium question came up in the running area, Adelle Davis had mentioned it in her book *Let's Eat Right to Keep Fit.* She says it has to be taken in correct combination with calcium to do much good. Miss Davis notes, "The correct proportion appears to be approximately twice as much calcium as magnesium, or 500 milligrams of magnesium for each 1000 milligrams of calcium." (The Recommended Daily Allowances for the two minerals are about 400 mg. magnesium and 800 mg. calcium.) Miss Davis adds that eating magnesium compounds without the needed calcium can produce symptoms of "muscular weakness, listlessness, lethargy, drowsiness, lack of coordination, speech difficulties, slow heartbeat, nausea and vomiting"—or worse. Runners are unlikely to get the "or worse" symptoms, but the others are serious enough to warrant attention.

The following foods have the highest magnesium content listed in milligrams per pound of the edible portion. The Recommended Daily Allowance of the mineral is 400 for a man in his early twenties. The average daily loss through the feces is 138 milligrams, but a runner may lose 50-100 percent more, as well as losing it through sweating.

Spinach, dehydrated	4,327	Curry powder	1,288
Cottonseed flour	2,948	Parsley, dried	1,284
Wheat bran, crude	2,223	Soybean flour, high-fat	1,234
Coffee, instant powder	2,068	Almonds, dried	1,225
Cocoa, dry powder	1,905	Cashew nuts	1,211
Wheat bran, cereal	1,095	Soybeans, dry seeds	1,202
Tea, instant powder	1,792	Molasses, blackstrap	1,170
Peanut flour, defatted	1,633	Soybean flour, full fat	1,120
Wheat germ	1,524	Yeast, brewers	1,048
Soybean flour, defatted	1,406	Cowpeas, dry seeds	1,043
Mustard, dried	1,343	Buckwheat, whole grain	1,039
Chocolate, bitter	1,325	Brazil nuts	1,021
Soybean flour, low-fat	1,311	Peanuts, raw	934

21
Extra Iron for Women

"Women have nearly twice the iron requirement of men." The line comes from an advertisement for an iron supplement, but it's more than a selling gimmick. The Food and Nutrition Board says the same thing. Women from puberty through menopause (about age 13 through late 40s) should get 18 milligrams of iron a day, while men need only 10 milligrams.

Iron is one of the most important substances in the body, appearing in every red blood cell. In the form of hemoglobin, it transports oxygen. And of course it keeps the runners running.

Writer and marathoner Janet Newman of Oregon has dug up facts linking iron deficiency with women's running capacities. She says research indicates that the average woman in the 20-30 age-group has 15 percent less hemoglobin than a man per 100 milliliters of blood. So women can carry far less than men. Many women, she notes, are chronically anemic—or have a low red blood cell count. The result is physical weakness, which causes obvious problems in running. Janet herself has this problem. She writes:

"I might add my own experiences with low hemoglobin counts. I seem to be chronically anemic but can remedy the situation with daily iron supplements and an emphasis on iron/protein in my diet. I have found a direct correlation between my running performances and my hemoglobin count. While doing about the same amount of training, all my best performances came when my hemoglobin was normal. When the hemoglobin count dropped to 48%, my running time slowed markedly—up to a minute per mile in races a mile to 13 miles long. Returning to iron pills, in one week the hemoglobin count rose 10% and I could feel a pronounced difference. My legs in particular lost their feeling of heaviness."

She advises other women who suspect they have anemia to take iron supplements and have regular blood tests. "Symptoms to watch for would be a general tired feeling, an unaccountable drop in performance, 'dead' legs and a pale complexion," Janet says.

Men can suffer from anemia, too, but women—because of their menstrual cycle—are much more susceptible. Individuals with anemic symptoms can take any number of iron pills or tonics available commercially. Geritol is one.

The following foods are naturally rich in iron. They're listed here with the milligram count per average serving.

Beef liver (2 oz.)	5.0 mg.	Chicken (½ breast)	1.3 mg.
Dried beans (¾ cup)	3.5 mg.	Egg (1 medium)	1.1 mg.
Beef pot roast (2 oz.)	2.9 mg.	Rice (¾ cup)	1.1 mg.
Pork chop (1 chop)	2.2 mg.	Tomato juice (4 oz.)	1.1 mg.
Spinach (½ cup)	2.0 mg.	Haddock (1 fillet)	1.0 mg.
Ham (2 oz.)	1.6 mg.	Macaroni (¾ cup)	1.0 mg.
Apricots (½ cup)	1.5 mg.	Bologna (2 slices)	1.0 mg.
Green peas (½ cup)	1.5 mg.	Sweet potato (1 med.)	1.0 mg.
Dried prunes (5 prunes)	1.5 mg.		

22
Vitamins to Run On
Ludvig Prokop, M.D.

Vitamin balance is related to physical—especially athletic—performance capacity. In all clinical cases of vitamin deficiency, the first symptom to appear is a reduction of physical capacity. And in hard work the need for various vitamins increases markedly, so that even with so-called normal doses a deficiency can result.

This means too that vitamins only produce a demonstrable and noticeable influence on performance when errors are made in composition and amounts in the diet. With a full-valued diet, if one adds even high amounts of additional vitamins, you can expect little positive effect.

There are great differences in the importance of individual vitamins for physical performance, and in optimal individual doses. In many aspects of vitamin effects we still lack legitimate, performance-specific, comparable, and placebo-tested results. We often must draw our conclusions from clinical studies.

With that introduction, I'll move on to discuss individual vitamins and their roles in athletics. Vitamin A, the B-complex, C, E, and P appear to be most important in endurance sports such as running, while vitamins D and K have no known effects on endurance capacity.

Vitamin A. Relatively little is known about the specific influence of vitamin A (*axerophtol*) on physical performance. It plays an important role in certain aging processes in connective tissue. A deficiency can provoke disturbances in sexual hormone metabolism and atrophy of the adrenal cortex. This has meaning for the mastery of performance demands because of the central position of the adrenals in the stress system. In high performance conditions, athletes should increase the intake of vitamin A to double the normal dose—i.e., they should take 3-4 milligrams per day.

Vitamin B-complex. Of the vitamin B group, vitamins B1, B2, niacin, and B12 seem performance-specific. In all vitamins of the B group, a decrease in spontaneous initiative and activity is one of the first deficiency symptoms.

1. *Vitamin B1 (thiamine)* is, in its physiologically effective form, necessary for the reduction of grape sugar (glucose or dextrose). Therefore, it is necessary for any increase in caloric use in all kinds of endurance performance. The daily requirement is 6-8 milligrams according to calories burned.

2. *Vitamin B2 (lactoflavin, riboflavin)* is also pertinent to endurance activity because of its importance in the formation of yellow respiratory enzyme. A normal daily requirement of 2-4 milligrams is indicated for high performance.

3. *Niacin (the PP factor)* is indispensable for the building and reduction of carbohydrates, as well as fats and proteins. For endurance performance, 40 milligrams—or double the normal requirement—is indicated.

4. *Vitamin B12* has an antianemic effect, plus specific effects on the metabolism of amino acids and the nervous system. Again, higher than normal doses are recommended, particularly for athletes performing at high altitudes.

Vitamin C. This vitamin (also called ascorbic acid) undoubtedly occupies a central position in connection with performance ability. This ubiquitous substance is partially responsible for the economy of almost all metabolic processes in the body. Ascorbic acid deficiency reduces physical performance capacity, and during physical exertion its underbalance is intensified. The vitamin C requirement of athletes and hard laborers is therefore significantly above the common norms. It may amount to 500 milligrams daily. This is especially true for endurance performance, particularly during severe weather.

However, vitamin C requirements are often irrationally exaggerated. During the Austrian bicycle tour, we found a daily elimination of vitamin C amounting to as much as four grams in the urine.

My own extensive investigations also have proved that vitamin C in the *natural* form (for example, in fruit juices) is clearly superior to synthetic ascorbic acid. We were able to objectify this in experiments with standardized stresses. The tests showed a decrease in oxygen debt and lowering of pulse and blood pressure. The reason for this increased effectiveness lies in the stabilization of vitamin C in fruit juices by the vitamin P group and other substances.

Vitamin E. Vitamin E (*topopherols*) assumes great importance for muscular performance capacity through an influence on circulation and capillarization, which improve utilization of oxygen. This gives vitamin E special significance in endurance performance.

As with vitamin C, natural vitamin E (for example, in wheat germ oil) has a certain superiority over equal dosages of synthetic vitamins.

Because of limited storage by the body, a continuous supply of perhaps 10-30 milligrams per day is necessary.

Vitamin P. The vitamin P-complex (*rutin, citrin, hesperidin*), used in relatively large amounts by the body, has a certain indirect influence on performance because of its stabilizing effect on vitamin C—as well as possibly other water-soluble vitamins.

The following chart summarizes average vitamin requirements for an athlete weighing 70 kilograms (154 pounds).

Vitamin	Nonathlete (mg.)	SPEED/STRENGTH		ENDURANCE	
		Training (mg.)	Racing (mg.)	Training (mg.)	Racing (mg.)
A	1.5	2	2-3	3	3-6
B$_1$	1.5	2-4	2-4	3-5	4-8
B$_2$	2	3	3	3-4	3-4
Niacin	20	30	30-40	30-40	40
C	70	100-140	140-200	140-200	200-240
E	7-10	14-20	24-30	20-30	30-50

Endurance capacity is often not so much a question of taking vitamins in high dosages, but assuring the simultaneous working of various vitamins in a physiologically balanced group—the way they are commonly found in nature. This is above all true of vitamins A, B_1, B_2, C, and E. An overdose of these vitamins, perhaps with the exception of vitamin E, can easily disturb the balance and thereby decrease performance capacity.

Therefore, multivitamin preparations as "means of building oneself up" during strenuous training and before competition seem more favorable than high dosages of individual vitamins.

The hubbub over vitamins has helped spread the opinion that one hardly needs to be concerned with real vitamin deficiencies any longer, and that the demand for an increase in vitamin values of food is exaggerated. However, there are alarming researches—even from economically well-situated countries—that contradict such optimistic views. For example, an investigation of U.S. teenagers concerning their intake of vitamin C showed only 10.3 percent of the boys and 52.4 percent of the girls reaching the standard recommendations of the Food and Nutrition Board. This is a result on the one hand of overeating carbohydrates, and on the other of increasing consumption of "practical" canned foods. It is obvious that during athletic stresses real inadequacies can result. The vitamin balance of the athlete for the present continues to demand special attention.

Part IV
The Body's Weight

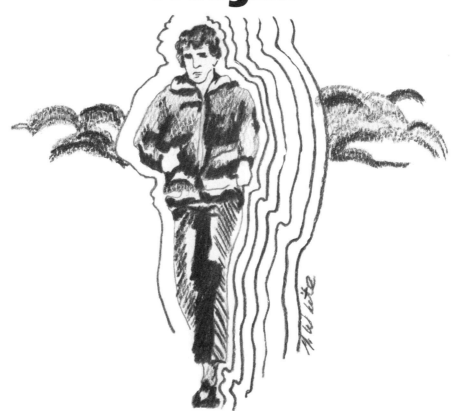

23
Getting More from Less

In 1925, a young German runner read Paavo Nurmi's statement, "All people eat too much and are therefore incapable of good performances." Ernst van Aaken never forgot what the Finnish runner said.

Van Aaken, now in his sixties, has made a lifelong study of running methods and nutrition (he talks about the two as one). His combined role of medical doctor and running coach has given him a unique perspective on these subjects. Van Aaken is a forceful, opinionated man. His ideas on training and eating are unorthodox, and acceptance of his thinking has come slowly—even in West Germany. His ideas rest on two principles:

1. running slowly to increase heart volume and oxygen intake

2. eating lightly to reduce body weight

The two are complementary, because the long slow running he recommends cuts the weight load, and lower body weight boosts heart efficiency. Van Aaken says the entire system operates better when it's lighter. By "lighter" he means considerably below normal weight. "One should eat so little," van Aaken says, "that he stays 10 to 20% under so-called normal weights." (See clarification of "normal" or "average" weights in the chapters that follow.)

Van Aaken offers a number of scientific reasons for his low-weight theory, as well as a mound of test data. But none of his reasons are as compelling to the runner/reader as actual experience on the track.

Here, van Aaken points to one of his students—Harald Norpoth. Norpoth has competed in the 1964, 1968, and 1972 Olympic Games and has held a number of European middle-distance records. He is 6'1" tall, and weighs just over 130. He obviously inherited a tendency toward thinness, but van Aaken's training and eating regimen no doubt pushed him down lower than he normally would be. This was lower, in fact, than many people would consider safe or healthy. Norpoth is van Aaken's idea of a classic runner: a strong motor inside a light frame. The idea, the doctor says, is to develop a powerful cardiovascular system capable of sucking in and using huge amounts of oxygen. The bigger a runner's heart volume is in relation to his body size, the more endurance he will have.

He explains: "The normal adult man has a heart volume of about 600 cubic centimeters. Sprinters have for the most part also only 600 cm.[3] Middle distance runners have a heart volume of 750-900 cm.[3], the long distance men have volumes of 900-1200 cm.[3], and many professional bicycle racers have heart volumes in excess of 1200 cm.[3] The largest hearts were found in professional cyclists, long distance rowers and marathon runners."

This is related to body weight.

> If one divides the heart volume, expressed in cubic centimeters, by the body weight, stated in kilograms, the result is what I have termed the "endurance quotient." I have found that the best long distance runners in the world show a quotient of 17, while very good—not the top—distance runners have at the very least a quotient betweeen 12 and 14.
>
> The astonishing thing, though, is that children 5-14 years of age whom I have examined have had much higher endurance quotients (often in the 12-14 range) on the average than untrained adults. The reason for this is that in relation to their body weight children have a greater capacity, especially if they are lively children. To use a technical expression derived from the automobile, they have a strong "heart motor" and a light "car body."

Ideally, van Aaken thinks, all endurance runners should cultivate this combination—high fuel supply and lowest possible cargo.

"Breathing," he says, "is more important than eating. Without breathing, man perishes within a few minutes, whereas he would be able to work 40 days consuming nothing but fruit juice and vegetable juice."

Breathing is easier, van Aaken claims, when weight is light, while extra weight puts an unneeded burden on the oxygen system. This is why he recommends reducing to at least 10 percent below average weight, and ideally 20 percent below. He says a runner needs 2,000 liters of oxygen to burn away one kilogram (2.2 pounds) of weight, estimating that this requires about 100 kilometers of running.

Runners who are light at the start, van Aaken says, can get by on less training mileage. According to him, the greatest value of big mileage is as a weight-reducer. "Their [the extra-long runs'] main effect on heavily built Peter Snell was to get his weight down. They should not be used to excess for slim runners like Norpoth and Bodo Tummler (bronze medalist in the 1968 Olympic 1500-meters)."

Van Aaken thinks light eating is a better way to lose weight than long running. He recommends minimal caloric intake and periodic fasting.

He says, "If you eat little and train down to a low body weight, you will save oxygen—something our theoretical dieticians have apparently not thought about. Expressed in calories, a marathon runner must very often undercut the basic 1,600 to 1,700 calorie level—regardless of training and occupation—because the organism is able to get along on a minimum.

"It is not eating that makes the master, nor a particular diet. Rather, it is eating very little of the diet, and running on an empty stomach, running on 'trained' reserves of many kinds."

Here's where fasting comes in. He has found that occasional fasts train the body to live on its own built-in resources. (It has the additional benefit of cutting weight.) "The middle and long distance runner of the future," he says, "must learn how to fast, the best thing being to run with a certain feeling of hunger. Digestion shortly before or during a race wastes energy."

Predictably, van Aaken comes out strongly against such practices as prerace carbohydrate "loading" and eating on the run.

Scientists recommend eating during the marathon, when it has been proven in practice that the best endurance results are achieved when one completely shuts off digestion during athletic activities and lives off reserves built up over a long time in training. It is therefore necessary to have fasted very often for at least 14 hours, in order to train the full distance with a completely empty stomach, so that carbohydrates are built up in the liver from reserves already present in the organism. Endurance activity can be carried on for days with almost no food, as was shown in a 500-kilometer walk in France in 1971.

When not fasting, van Aaken says, "A runner may eat anything he likes and what is customarily offered in his social surroundings. But he should not go beyond 2,000 calories per day." He adds, "Only the athlete who runs daily, lives modestly and eats little but well will ever become a good runner."

Almost 50 years later, the Paavo Nurmi influence is still there.

24
Finding the Ideal Weight

Finding the best body weight isn't easy. One way is to labor through a long trial-and-error process, checking results at different levels. This takes time. Another is to check a medical weight chart. This almost invariably will be too high. Another is to have a doctor measure your fat percentage. This is expensive. There is no simple way to determine one's best weight—the level representing maximum strength with minimum extra baggage. Ideal weight is unique to the individual, based on body makeup, and the physical work one is trying to accomplish. A heavily muscled, thick-boned man is naturally going to have a higher ideal weight than a light-bodied ectomorph. A sprinter, taking powerful bursts of effort, needs more muscle bulk than a distance runner gliding his miles. No single weight chart can suit them all.

At best, any formula is a generalization requiring individual interpretation. There are formulas, however, that give ideal weights with fair accuracy. One formula, published in *Runner's World,* is not particularly accurate. That one indicates that the best weight for a distance runner is twice his height in inches. For instance, if a runner is 5'7" (or 67 inches) tall, he should weigh 134 pounds. This is fine—if you happen to be 5'7" tall. Otherwise, the formula is a gross oversimplification. The farther one gets from 5'7", the less accurate the formula.

Jack Bachelor is 6' 6 5/8" tall. Under the height-doubled system, Bachelor should weight 157 pounds. One of Jack's training partners pointed out—correctly—that "if he weighed 157 pounds, you wouldn't be able to see him." Bachelor might end up in the hospital if he reduced that severely. On the other hand, a 5'5" runner has it too easy. He might actually be pudgy around the middle at 130 pounds.

We need a better formula than that—one that is fair to people at the extreme heights. Medical doctor and author Irwin Maxwell Stillman has one that may be the best available. Dr. Stillman takes a somewhat unorthodox, yet apparently highly successful, approach to weight reduction. Besides treating thousands of overweight patients, he has written two books—*The Doctor's Quick Weight Loss Diet* and *The Inches-Off Diet.* Some of his suggestions appear later in this chapter, but here our main concern is with the formula.

Stillman tells how to figure "average" weight for an individual's weight and height.

1. Men start with 110 pounds and 5 feet. For every inch above that height, add 5½ pounds. If a man is 6'0" tall, he adds 66 pounds (12 x 5½ = 66) to 110 pounds. His average weight is 176 pounds.

2. Women start with 100 pounds (not 110) and 5 feet. For every extra inch, add 5 (not 5½) pounds. A 5'5" woman adds 25 pounds (5 x 5 = 25) to 100 pounds. Her average weight is 125 pounds.

This isn't the end of it, though. There are two more catches.

1. In theory, people stop growing in their early twenties. Stillman says no one should ever weigh more than he did at age 25. People under 25 subtract one pound per year from their average weight, down to age 18. (If the 6'0" male is only 20 years old, his average drops to 171 pounds.) The formula doesn't apply to rapidly growing children under 18.

2. Average weights are just a starting point. Stillman writes, "I don't believe we should be guided by average weights. They are often too high because Americans are generally overweight." He says the ideal weight is 10 percent below the average for one's height and age. (The 20-year-old, 6'0" male's ideal weight, then, is 154 pounds.)

Dr. Stillman further recommends, "If you're an athlete it is best to weigh about five pounds less than the ideal weight listed."

This formula is more fair than the old height-doubled idea. With it, Jack Bachelor sees he's really 15 pounds or so below his "ideal" weight. The smug short guy finally sees he isn't as skinny as he thought.

RUNNERS' WEIGHT CHARTS

To save all the figuring, here is Stillman's weight formula in chart form. First, for men use 100 pounds and 5 feet as a base and add 5½ pounds for each additional inch. For women, use 100 pounds and 5 feet as base figures, and add 5 pounds for each additional inch. (Deduct 1 pound for each year under 25, down to age 18.)

These calculations give *average* weight. Subtract 10% of that for Stillman's *ideal* weight; subtract 20% for the distance runner's ideal recommended by Ernst van Aaken. (Weights here are rounded to the nearest pound.)

MEN'S WEIGHTS

Height	Ave.	-10%	-20%	Height	Ave.	-10%	-20%
5' 0" (60")	110	99	88	5' 9" (69")	160	144	128
5' 1" (61")	116	104	93	5' 10" (70")	165	149	132
5' 2" (62")	121	109	97	5' 11" (71")	171	154	137
5' 3" (63")	127	114	101	6' 0" (72")	176	159	141
5' 4" (64")	132	119	106	6' 1" (73")	182	164	145
5' 5" (65")	138	124	110	6' 2" (74")	186	168	149
5' 6" (66")	143	129	115	6' 3" (75")	192	173	153
5' 7" (67")	149	134	119	6' 4" (76")	197	178	158
5' 8" (68")	154	139	123	6' 5" (77")	203	182	162

WOMEN'S WEIGHTS

Height	Ave.	-10%	-20%	Height	Ave.	-10%	-20%
5' 0" (60")	100	90	80	5' 6" (66")	130	117	104
5' 1" (61")	105	95	84	5' 7" (67")	135	122	108
5' 2" (62")	110	99	88	5' 8" (68")	140	126	112
5' 3" (63")	115	104	92	5' 9" (69")	145	131	116
5' 4" (64")	120	108	96	5' 10" (70")	150	135	120
5' 5" (65")	125	113	100	5' 11" (71")	155	140	124

25
Longer
and Lighter

You don't often see obese runners, and only rarely do you
see any runners heavy-boned or heavy-muscled enough to
push their weight above the so-called average for their height.
Average weight for the general population tends to be around
the upper limit, except for a few sprinters.

Earlier in this part, Dr. Stillman offered a workable
formula for figuring average weights. He said that 10 percent
below that average is "ideal." Dr. van Aaken said that a distance runner should reduce to 20 percent below average. We
checked out these recommendations on the basis of what leading runners actually weigh, and the height-weight figures are
close to Stillman's and van Aaken's ideals.

The analysis involved about 300 of the top American male
runners—the best 10-30 athletes in each of the running events
for 1972. *Track & Field News* supplied the height-weight data.
Stillman's weight formula (see preceding chapter) is the basis
for the calculations.

Preliminary checks indicated that sprinters are heaviest and
runners get progressively lighter as they go up in distance—
marathoners being lightest. This fact is based on physiological
principles. Faster, more explosive, runs require greater muscle
power and bulk, and less total energy expenditure; longer runs
use leaner endurance muscles, and continuous effort burns up
more calories. Thin runners gravitate toward the longer distances, and the act of running long makes them leaner yet.

Let's go to the comparative figures, and see if this is indeed
how it works, and to what extent. Heights for all runners,
regardless of event, average about the same—about 5'11" except for hurdlers. Obviously, the best hurdlers need long legs.
They are, as a group, about two inches taller than the runners.
In weight:

1. Sprinters (100-440 yards) are the heaviest of the runners—but they are still a bit lighter than the average man. The typical sprinter in this sample is 23 years old, 5'11", and 163 pounds. He's 2½ percent lighter than average for his height and age.

2. Hurdlers (120-yard highs and 440-yard intermediates) are considerably lighter than sprinters running comparable distances. The typical 23-year-old, 6'11" hurdler weighs 168 pounds—or about 6 percent below average.

3. Middle-distance runners (880 yards to six miles) are lighter yet. As a group, they're well below Stillman's "ideal," with a combined percentage 12 percent under normal. Middle-distance men's average is 23, height 5' 10½", weight 147.

4. Long-distance runners (above the track distances) are the lightest of all. At 15 percent below normal, they're edging toward van Aaken's "ideal." The average marathoner is 25 years old, 5' 10½", and 142 pounds.

5. Walkers (20 and 50 kilometers) are somewhat heavier than their distance-running counterparts. At age 30, 5'11", and 153 pounds, they average 10 percent below normal.

The accompanying chart breaks down the figures by event—100, 220, etc. The trend to lighter weight for longer distances is just as pronounced here.

Overall, the best weight for sprinters seems to be somewhere between the average for an individual's height and age and perhaps 10 percent below. In this study, an equal number of 100-yard sprinters are slightly above and below average. A few of the "overweights" hang on in the 220, a smaller percentage yet appear in the 440 and hurdles, and only one above-average man showed up in the 880 and mile. From there up, there are none.

The heaviest concentration of sprinters and hurdlers are in the average to minus-10 percent category. This area accounts for about 7 men in every 10. At the 880, however, the emphasis shifts. This is the start of endurance running. Each step up from there, an increasing majority of runners weigh 10 to 20 percent below average. A significant number of runners (one in five marathoners) are lighter than 20 percent. The message is clear. Weight is definitely related to running performance—increasingly important as distance goes up. It is extremely rare in races above a half-mile to see a runner of even "average" weight. The normal man's average weight is the runner's obesity level. Runners have a lower set of weight standards because their performance standards are higher.

EVENT-BY-EVENT MEASUREMENTS

This chart is based on data from the leading U.S. male runners during the 1972 season—about 300 athletes in all. The right-hand column is the most important one. It lists how far below average the weights of runners are in each event. Only in the 100 are the weights average; the rest are well below.

EVENT	AGE	HEIGHT	WEIGHT	% BELOW
Sprints				
100	23.0	5' 10.0"	163.3	—
220	22.7	5' 10.7"	161.5	3.3%
440	23.1	5' 11.6"	165.2	3.7%
Hurdles				
Highs	22.5	6' 1.5"	174.6	3.8%
Intermediates	23.3	6' 0.7"	163.4	8.5%
Middle Distances				
880	22.5	6' 0.3"	157.2	10.4%
Mile	22.7	5' 11.0"	149.1	12.0%
3 miles	23.6	5' 10.4"	146.0	12.3%
6 miles	24.6	5' 10.1"	143.0	12.8%
Steeplechase	23.3	5' 10.8"	143.7	14.2%
Long Distance				
Marathon	25.6	5' 10.3"	142.0	15.0%
Race Walks				
20 kilometers	30.4	5' 11.2"	153.6	11.0%
50 kilometers	29.8	5' 10.7"	152.3	10.0%

26
New Weight-Watchers

Weight-watching is the great American pastime. Like the weather, everyone talks about weight, but most people don't do much to change it. Runners can't afford just to talk about theirs, however, because weight is particularly critical to them. If it slips outside the narrow boundaries of the ideal range, their performance reflects it. They have to put weight where they think it belongs, and then watch that it stays there. In this sense, the runner's scales are as important to him as his stopwatch. A daily weight record is as valuable as a daily mileage tally.

Running weight-watching is tricky for several reasons. Here are a number of points to keep in mind. Some are suggestions; some are warnings.

Decide on an ideal weight. The Stillman-van Aaken formulas offer good starting points, but they have to be tempered by your personal situation. Listen to the lessons of your own experience. That will help you find your personal ideal.

Get to that ideal weight. If you're not there already, chances are you're on the high side. There are lots of ways to get down—all of which involve work and/or sacrifice; running more and/or eating less. Dr. Stillman advises, "Eat to satisfy your hunger, not to pamper your appetite. . . . You're better off eating smaller meals six times a day than three bigger meals as is the general custom."

Lose gradually. The only successful diets are those that modify overall eating habits and are fairly easy to carry on for periods of months and years. Drastic, quick-loss schemes are often self-defeating because (a) they're hard to stick with, and (b) they may disrupt internal equilibrium and drag down performance.

Keep a record. Weigh yourself every day, at the same time, and under the same conditions. An easy system to follow is to weigh yourself first thing in the morning, after you've gone to the bathroom, and before you've put on clothes, run, or had breakfast. Write the weight alongside the record of everyday running.

Don't be fooled by false losses. "False" losses are liquid drains. A runner can easily lose four or five pounds of sweat a day by running. In a year's time, he may sweat away a half-ton of weight. Obviously, this is a temporary loss, lasting only as long as it takes to do some heavy drinking. The liquid losses needn't concern you unless they show up the next morning in a 2-3 pound weight drop. Sudden drops like this are symptoms of chronic dehydration.

Watch for creeping gains. Weight doesn't usually accumulate overnight. Such gains are easy enough to handle if they do occur. The hard ones to catch are the ones you hardly notice. A few extra calories a day may add no more than a few ounces a month, but over a year's time these ounces multiply into pounds. You wake up one morning five years later and realize you've gained 10 pounds. Here again daily weight-watching is invaluable. Dr. Stillman says, "Any time you see that scale mark three pounds more than your desired weight, consider it more serious than if your thermometer showed three degrees or more over your normal temperature."

Running isn't an invitation to gluttony. The runner doesn't inherit a license to eat. The sport burns up a hundred or so calories a mile; an hour's run uses around a thousand. It takes about 3,500 calories to lose a pound, and the same to gain one. A milkshake can cancel out the weight-losing effect of an hour's run.

Runners have efficient systems. As they get into better and better condition, the body "idles" at a lower rate than the average person's. The effect is that a runner burns a bundle of calories while running, but uses a lot fewer to survive the rest of the day. Therefore, he may not need gross amounts of food.

Stay out of the vicious cycle. This starts with thinking a higher-than-ideal weight is the best one. Running reduces your ideal weight. You eat heavier to push it back up. The body works harder to get it back down. You eat; you strain. Van Aaken says one of the main reasons for super-long training is to reduce weight. If the weight is already low, you're already halfway there—without so much long, hard running.

This isn't kid's stuff. Little of the information in this chapter applies directly to growing children. They need plenty of food to grow on, and shouldn't be restricted unless they're obviously fat. Young children and teenagers who run probably are so light already that none of this need concern them. Dr. George Sheehan agrees with van Aaken that young children are the greatest natural runners. Sheehan writes of a preteenager:

> He is pound for pound the world's best endurance athlete. And he moves with the grace and elegance of the free animal. Strength and power he may not have, but fatigue is foreign to him. This is because he has the biggest heart volume for his weight that he will ever have unless he is an Olympic champion. He is therefore the nearest thing to perpetual motion in human form you will ever see, and yet at other times he is capable of the contented lethargy of a lion after a kill.

Both the perpetual motion and contented lethargy vanish gradually with age—and added weight. The point where he quits growing up and starts spreading out is the critical one. Stillman's weight calculations begin at age 18, and he says no one should gain another pound after age 25. Between 18 and 25 is when the gap between ideal and reality begins to show and spread.

27
Fast, Faster, Fastest
Gary Chilton

In 1968, I took some positive action. I tossed out my cigarettes, began a weight-loss diet, and started jogging. Today, four years later and 45 pounds lighter, I am the proud owner of a couple of sub-three-hour marathons. During my four-year journey from sickness to health, I have had experiences with diet and weight control that may be of value to other runners who have had to fight the battle of the bulge. As a result of my experience with training, special diets, and fasting, I am convinced the greatest single limiting factor in successful long-distance running is body weight.

This does not imply that training is unimportant. I am merely suggesting that optimum training and improvement can take place when the runner is at his "ideal" weight. In other words, if a runner is carrying 10 or 15 pounds of excess baggage in the form of fatty tissue, and continues to consume enough calories to maintain this excess, then no amount of running training can bring about an optimum performance level. On the other hand, dramatic and almost instantaneous improvement in running performances can be noted even on reduced mileage when proper attention is given to diet and weight control.

I offer my own case history as an example. I began reducing from 185 pounds. The height/weight charts indicated an average weight of around 155 pounds for my 5'10" medium frame. With a balanced, but reduced, calorie diet and a daily four-mile jog, I was able to lose the indicated 30 pounds within a few months. According to my doctor, I was in excellent health and my weight was just right for my build. At the time, I had no reason to doubt the doctor's observation. At 155 pounds, I felt better than I had in years and my casual jogging had developed into competitive long-distance running.

For almost three years, I trained and raced at 155 pounds. My training was almost exclusively slow continuous running— sometimes 80 and 100 miles a week. Improvement was slow. Also, I concluded that 3:20 marathons were about the best a 34-year-old ex-fat guy should expect on three years' training. I was beginning to think running wasn't worth the effort. About that time, I read about Ernst van Aaken, who advocated—among other things—drastic weight reduction for long-distance runners. According to Dr. van Aaken's recommendations, I should weigh between 130 and 140 pounds—a far cry from my comfortable 155 pounds. Dr. van Aaken also recommended occasional days of strict fasting in order to train the body to live on reserves. The recommendation seemed to make a lot of sense so I decided to experiment.

I started with a three-day fast during which I drank only small quantities of orange juice, vegetable juice, and unsweetened tea. Training during this period was eight miles per day at about an eight-minute-mile pace. This first attempt at fasting was unpleasant, to say the least. I was uncomfortable, hungry, and my running was strained. In spite of the discomfort, the fast was effective in removing about six pounds.

For the next few weeks, I followed a program of fasting one day a week and restricting my intake to less than 2,000 calories on the remaining days. Within three weeks, I had lost about 15 pounds and I began to notice a dramatic improvement in training performance, as well as an unusual sense of lightness, agility, and overall well-being.

During this weight-loss program, I maintained an average of about 60 miles per week of easy running. I was chopping minutes off my training loops with absolutely no increase in effort. A loop that had been difficult to run in less than 1:45 suddenly became an easy effort at 1:35. Another loop that had been a strain to cover in less than 1:22 suddenly became a relaxed 1:15 effort. A one-hour loop became a 50-minute loop. I was training at a pace between 30 seconds and a minute per mile faster than three short weeks before—and I was doing it with less effort!

The decrease in running effort was accompanied by other

indications of increased capacity. Within a one-week period, my resting heart rate, which had been 48 for two years, fell to 42. I noted an increased ability to withstand heat, as well as an increased capacity for running uphill. The weight loss alone was responsible for this increased training capacity, since I had made no other changes in diet or routine.

Increased training performance has also been reflected in improved racing times. An eight-mile course that took 52:32 to cover two years ago, I have recently covered in 46:47. A marathon course that took 3:33 two years ago has been improved to 2:57. I have only trained a short while at this new level of fitness, and I am looking forward to continued improvement.

I attribute my improved training and racing performances to weight loss accomplished through strict fasting. The reduction in weight allows me to tolerate a greater level of training without increased effort. Maintaining a lower weight also allows a great degree of freshness to be retained while running "quality" workouts. Increased tolerance for heat reduces overall stress and makes workouts more enjoyable. Without the extra weight, I'm running less and enjoying it more.

Of course, a lot of runners don't have a real weight problem, but I'm willing to bet that a good percentage are carrying more than they need for optimum performance. It's all too easy to tell ourselves that our running alone will keep us at the proper weight. This kind of reasoning is an automatic license to eat everything in sight.

Sometimes an illness or injury forces a layoff and we don't give proper attention to adjusting intake. A person with the metabolism and appetite of a distance runner can blow up like the Goodyear Blimp with a few weeks of inactivity. Just a few pounds of fat can make a big difference in running performance. If your running has been at a standstill for awhile and you haven't been on the scale lately, maybe you have accumulated some excess baggage.

Check yourself. If you aren't 10-20 percent below what the standard height/weight charts recommend, maybe a weight reduction would give you that shot in the arm you've been waiting for. Travel light. It makes a difference.

Appendix

FOOD VALUES

DAIRY PRODUCTS

	Measure	Weight grams	Food Energy cal.	Protein grams	Fat grams	Carbohydrate grams	Calcium mg.	Potassium mg.	Vitamin B2 mg.	Vitamin B1 mg.	Vitamin B6 mg.	Vitamin C mg.
CHEESE												
Cheddar, shredded	1 cup	113	455	28	37	1	815	111	0.03	0.42	0.1	0
Cottage cheese	1 cup	225	235	28	10	6	135	190	0.05	0.37	0.3	Trace
Cream cheese	1 oz.	28	100	2	10	—	—	34	Trace	0.06	Trace	0
Pasteurized American cheese	1 oz.	28	105	6	6	Trace	174	46	0.01	0.10	Trace	0
CREAM												
Half-and-half	1 tbsp.	15	20	Trace	2	1	16	19	0.01	0.02	Trace	Trace
Cream, sour	1 tbsp.	12	25	Trace	3	1	14	17	Trace	0.02	Trace	Trace
MILK												
Whole	1 cup	244	150	8	8	11	291	370	0.09	0.40	0.2	2
Lowfat (2%)	1 cup	244	120	8	5	12	297	377	0.10	0.40	0.2	2
Nonfat (skim)	1 cup	245	85	8	Trace	12	302	406	0.09	0.37	0.2	2
ICE CREAM												
Hardened	1 cup	133	270	5	115	32	176	257	0.05	0.33	0.1	1
Soft (frozen custard)	1 cup	173	375	7	23	38	236	338	0.08	0.45	0.2	1
YOGURT												
Fruit-flavored	8 oz.	227	230	10	3	42	343	439	0.08	0.40	0.2	1

Plain	8 oz.	227	145	12	4	16	415	531	0.10	0.49	0.3	2
EGGS												
Fried in butter	1 egg	46	85	5	6	1	26	58	0.03	0.13	Trace	0
Hard-cooked, shell removed	1 egg	50	80	6	6	1	28	65	0.04	0.14	Trace	0
Scrambled (milk added) in butter; also omelet	1 egg	64	95	6	7	1	47	85	0.04	0.16	Trace	0
FATS AND OILS												
Butter	1 tbsp.	14	100	Trace	12	Trace	3	4	Trace	Trace	Trace	0
Vegetable shortening	1 tbsp.	13	110	0	13	0	0	0	0	0	0	0
Margarine	1 tbsp.	14	100	Trace	12	Trace	0	4	Trace	Trace	Trace	0
Corn oil	1 tbsp.	14	120	0	14	0	0	0	0	0	0	0
Soybean-cottonseed oil blend, hydrogenated	1 tbsp.	14	120	0	14	0	0	0	0	0	0	0
FISH, MEAT, AND POULTRY												
FISH												
Haddock, breaded, fried	3 oz.	85	140	17	5	5	34	296	0.03	0.06	2.7	2
Ocean perch, breaded, fried	1 fillet	85	95	16	11	6	28	242	0.10	0.10	1.6	—
Tuna, canned (in oil, drained)	3 oz.	85	170	24	7	0	7	—	0.04	0.10	10.1	—
MEAT												
Bacon, broiled or fried, crisp	2 slices	15	85	4	8	Trace	2	35	0.08	0.05	0.8	—
Beef, braised, simmered, or roasted	3 oz.	85	245	23	16	0	10	184	0.04	0.18	3.6	—
Ground beef, broiled	2.9 oz.	82	235	20	17	0	9	221	0.07	0.17	4.4	—
Roast, oven cooked	3 oz.	85	375	17	33	0	8	189	0.05	0.13	3.1	—
Steak, sirloin, broiled	3 oz.	85	330	20	27	0	9	220	0.05	0.15	4.0	—

| Measure | Weight | Food Energy | Protein | Fat | Carbohydrate | Calcium | Potassium | Vitamin B2 | Vitamin B1 | Vitamin B6 | Vitamin C |
	cal.	grams	grams	grams	mg.	mg.	mg.	mg.	mg.	mg.	mg.
Lamb											
Chop, broiled — 3.1 oz.	89	360	18	32	0	8	200	0.11	0.19	4.1	—
Leg, roasted — 3 oz.	85	235	22	16	0	9	241	0.13	0.23	4.7	—
Liver, fried — 3 oz.	85	195	22	9	5	9	323	0.22	3.56	14.0	23
Ham, roasted — 3 oz.	85	245	18	19	0	8	199	0.40	0.15	3.1	—
Pork											
Chop — 2.7 oz.	78	305	19	25	0	9	216	0.75	0.22	4.5	—
Roast, oven cooked — 3 oz.	85	310	21	24	0	9	233	0.78	0.22	4.8	—
Sausages											
Bologna — 1 slice	28	85	3	8	Trace	2	65	0.05	0.06	0.7	—
Brown and serve — 1 link	17	70	3	6	Trace	—	—	—	—	—	—
Frankfurter, cooked — 1 ea.	56	170	7	15	1	3	—	0.08	0.11	1.4	—
Pork link, cooked — 1 link	13	60	2	6	Trace	1	35	0.10	0.04	0.5	—
Salami, cooked type — 1 slice	28	90	5	7	Trace	3	—	0.07	0.07	1.2	—
Veal, cutlet — 3 oz.	85	185	23	9	0	9	258	0.06	0.21	4.6	—
POULTRY											
Chicken, cooked											
Drumstick, fried — 1.3 oz.	38	90	12	4	Trace	6	—	0.03	0.15	2.7	—
Half-broiler, broiled — 6.2 oz.	176	240	42	7	0	16	483	0.09	0.35	15.5	—

Turkey, roasted, flesh without skin											
Dark meat	4 pcs.	85	175	26	7	0	—	338	0.03	0.20	3.6	—
Light meat	2 pcs.	85	150	28	3	0	—	349	0.04	0.12	9.4	—

FRUITS AND FRUIT PRODUCTS

Apples, raw, unpeeled	1 ea.	138	80	Trace	1	20	10	152	0.04	0.03	0.1	6
Apricots											
Raw	3	107	55	1	Trace	14	18	301	0.03	0.04	0.6	11
Canned	1 cup	258	220	2	Trace	57	28	604	0.05	0.05	1.0	10
Avocados, raw, whole	1 ea.	216	370	5	37	13	22	1303	0.24	0.43	3.5	30
Banana	1 ea.	119	100	1	Trace	26	10	440	0.06	0.07	0.8	12
Grapefruit, medium	1/2 ea.	241	50	1	Trace	13	20	166	0.05	0.02	0.2	44
Grapes, seedless	10	50	35	Trace	Trace	9	6	87	0.03	0.02	0.2	2
Lemonade, diluted	1 cup	248	105	Trace	Trace	28	2	40	0.01	0.02	0.2	17
Melons											
Cantaloupe	1/2 ea.	477	80	2	Trace	20	38	682	0.11	0.08	1.6	90
Honeydew	1/10 ea.	226	50	1	Trace	11	21	374	0.06	0.04	0.9	34
Oranges	1 ea.	131	65	1	Trace	16	54	263	0.13	0.05	0.5	66
Orange juice, frozen, diluted	1 cup	249	120	2	Trace	29	25	503	0.23	0.03	0.9	120
Papayas, raw	1 cup	140	55	1	Trace	14	28	328	0.06	0.06	0.4	78
Peaches, whole	1 ea.	100	40	1	Trace	10	9	202	0.02	0.05	1.0	7
Pears, raw, with skin, cored	1 ea.	164	100	1	1	25	13	213	0.03	0.07	0.2	7
Pineapple											
Raw, diced	1 cup	155	80	1	Trace	21	26	226	0.14	0.05	0.3	26
Canned	1 slice	105	80	Trace	Trace	20	12	101	0.08	0.02	0.2	7
Pineapple juice, unsweetened	1 cup	250	140	1	Trace	34	38	373	0.13	0.05	0.5	80
Raisins, seedless	1 cup	145	420	4	Trace	112	90	1106	0.16	0.12	0.7	1

	Measure	Weight	Food Energy	Protein	Fat	Carbohydrate	Calcium	Potassium	Vitamin B2	Vitamin B1	Vitamin B6	Vitamin C
	grams	cal.	grams	grams	grams	mg.	mg.	mg.	mg.	mg.	mg.	mg.
Strawberries, raw, whole berries	1 cup	149	55	1	1	13	31	244	0.04	0.10	0.9	88

GRAIN PRODUCTS

BREADS

	Measure	Weight	Food Energy	Protein	Fat	Carbohydrate	Calcium	Potassium	Vitamin B2	Vitamin B1	Vitamin B6	Vitamin C
Cracked-wheat bread	1 slice	25	65	2	1	13	22	34	0.08	0.06	0.08	Trace
French, enriched	1 slice	35	100	3	1	19	15	32	0.14	0.08	1.2	Trace
Rye bread	1 slice	25	60	2	Trace	13	19	36	0.07	0.05	0.7	0
White bread, enriched	1 slice	23	65	2	1	12	22	28	0.09	0.06	0.8	Trace
Whole-wheat bread	1 slice	25	60	3	1	12	25	68	0.06	0.03	0.7	Trace

BREAKFAST CEREALS

	Measure	Weight	Food Energy	Protein	Fat	Carbohydrate	Calcium	Potassium	Vitamin B2	Vitamin B1	Vitamin B6	Vitamin C
Oatmeal or rolled oats	1 cup	240	130	5	2	23	22	146	0.19	0.05	0.2	0
Bran flakes (40% bran)	1 cup	35	105	4	1	28	19	137	0.41	0.49	4.1	12
Cornflakes	1 cup	25	95	2	Trace	21	—	30	0.29	0.35	2.9	9
Wheat, puffed	1 cup	15	55	2	Trace	12	4	51	0.08	0.03	1.2	0
Wheat, shredded, plain biscuit	1	25	90	2	1	20	11	87	0.06	0.03	1.1	0

OTHER GRAIN PRODUCTS

	Measure	Weight	Food Energy	Protein	Fat	Carbohydrate	Calcium	Potassium	Vitamin B2	Vitamin B1	Vitamin B6	Vitamin C
Wheat germ	1 tbsp.	6	25	2	1	3	3	57	0.11	0.05	0.3	1
Cornmeal, whole-ground	1 cup	122	435	11	5	90	24	346	0.46	0.13	2.4	0
Crackers												
Graham	2	14	55	1	1	10	6	55	0.02	0.08	0.5	0

Saltines	4	11	50	1		8	2	13	0.05	0.05	0.4	0
Macaroni, enriched, cooked	1 cup	140	155	5		32	11	85	0.20	0.11	1.5	0
Pancakes (4-in. diam.)	1 cake	27	60	2		9	58	42	0.04	0.06	0.2	Trace
Rice, white, enriched	1 cup	205	225	4		50	21	57	0.23	0.02	2.1	0
Barley (pearled, light, uncooked)	1 cup	200	700	16		158	32	320	0.24	0.10	6.2	0
Wheat flour												
Sifted	1 cup	115	420	12		88	18	109	0.74	0.46	6.1	0
Whole wheat	1 cup	120	400	16		85	49	444	0.66	0.14	5.2	0

LEGUMES (DRY), NUTS, AND SEEDS

Almonds, shelled	1 cup	130	775	24	70	25	304	1005	0.31	1.20	4.6	Trace
Beans, cooked												
Great northern	1 cup	180	210	14	1	38	90	749	0.25	0.13	1.3	0
Navy	1 cup	190	225	15	1	40	95	790	0.27	0.13	1.3	0
Lima, cooked, drained	1 cup	190	230	16	1	49	55	1163	0.25	0.11	1.3	—
Coconut meat, fresh	1 cup	80	275	3	28	8	10	205	0.04	0.02	0.4	2
Lentils, whole, cooked	1 cup	200	210	16	Trace	39	50	498	0.14	0.12	1.2	0
Peanuts, roasted in oil, salted	1 cup	144	840	37	72	27	107	971	0.46	0.19	24.8	0
Peanut butter	1 tbsp.	16	95	4	8	3	9	100	0.02	0.02	2.4	0
Peas, split, dry, cooked	1 cup	200	230	16	1	42	22	592	0.30	0.18	1.8	—

SUGARS

Honey	1 tbsp.	21	65	Trace	0	17	1	11	Trace	0.01	0.1	Trace
Sugars												
Brown	1 cup	220	820	0	0	212	187	757	0.02	0.07	0.4	0
White	1 cup	200	770	0	0	199	0	6	0	0	0	0

VEGETABLES

	Measure grams	Weight cal.	Food Energy grams	Protein grams	Fat grams	Carbohydrate mg.	Calcium mg.	Potassium mg.	Vitamin B2 mg.	Vitamin B1 mg.	Vitamin B6 mg.	Vitamin C mg.
Asparagus, cooked	1 cup	145	30	3	Trace	5	30	265	0.23	0.26	2.0	38
Beans												
Lima, frozen, cooked, drained,	1 cup	180	210	13	Trace	40	63	709	0.16	0.09	2.2	22
Green, cooked, drained, from raw	1 cup	125	30	2	Trace	7	63	189	0.09	0.11	0.6	15
Bean sprouts, cooked, drained	1 cup	125	35	4	Trace	7	21	195	0.11	0.13	0.9	8
Beets, cooked, drained, peeled, whole 2 in. diam.	2 ea.	100	30	1	Trace	7	14	208	0.03	0.04	0.3	6
Broccoli, cooked, drained												
Fresh	1 cup	155	40	5	Trace	7	136	414	0.14	0.31	1.2	140
Frozen, chopped	1 cup	185	50	5	1	9	100	392	0.11	0.22	0.9	105
Brussels sprouts, cooked, drained	1 cup	155	55	7	1	10	50	423	0.12	0.22	1.2	135
Cabbage												
Raw	1 cup	90	20	1	Trace	5	44	210	0.05	0.05	0.3	42
Cooked, drained	1 cup	145	30	2	Trace	6	64	236	0.06	0.06	0.4	48
Carrots												
Raw	1 ea.	72	30	1	Trace	7	27	246	0.04	0.04	0.4	6
Cooked, drained	1 cup	155	50	1	Trace	11	51	344	0.08	0.08	0.8	9
Cauliflower												
Raw	1 cup	115	31	3	Trace	6	29	339	0.13	0.12	0.8	90

Food	Amount											
Cooked from raw	1 cup	125	30	3	Trace	5	26	258	0.11	0.10	0.8	69
Cooked from frozen	1 cup	180	30	3	Trace	6	31	373	0.07	0.09	0.7	74
Celery	1 stalk	40	5	Trace	Trace	2	16	136	0.01	0.01	0.1	4
Corn												
Cooked from raw	1 ear	140	70	2	1	16	2	151	0.09	0.08	1.1	7
Cooked from frozen	1 cup	165	130	5	1	31	5	304	0.15	0.10	2.5	8
Canned, cream style	1 cup	256	210	5	2	51	8	248	0.08	0.13	2.6	13
Canned, whole kernel	1 cup	210	175	5	1	43	6	204	0.06	0.13	2.3	11
Cucumber	6 large	28	5	Trace	Trace	1	7	45	0.01	0.01	0.1	3
Lettuce												
Butter, leaves	2	15	Trace	Trace	Trace	Trace	5	40	0.01	0.01	Trace	1
Iceberg pieces	1 cup	55	5	Trace	Trace	2	11	96	0.03	0.03	0.2	3
Mushrooms, raw	1 cup	70	20	2	Trace	3	4	290	0.07	0.32	2.9	2
Onions												
Raw, chopped	1 cup	170	65	3	Trace	15	46	267	0.05	0.07	0.3	17
Cooked	1 cup	210	60	3	Trace	14	50	231	0.06	0.06	0.4	15
Green	6 ea.	30	15	Trace	Trace	3	12	69	0.02	0.01	0.1	8
Peas, green												
Canned whole	1 cup	170	150	8	1	29	44	163	0.15	0.10	1.4	14
Frozen	1 cup	160	110	8	Trace	19	30	216	0.43	0.14	2.7	21
Potatoes												
Baked	1 ea.	156	145	4	Trace	33	14	782	0.15	0.07	2.7	31
Boiled	1 ea.	135	90	3	Trace	20	8	385	0.12	0.05	1.6	22
Pumpkin, canned	1 cup	245	80	2	1	19	61	588	0.07	0.12	1.5	12
Radishes, raw	4 ea.	18	5	Trace	Trace	1	5	58	0.01	0.01	0.1	5

	Measure	Weight	Food Energy	Protein	Fat	Carbohydrate	Calcium	Potassium	Vitamin B2	Vitamin B1	Vitamin B6	Vitamin C
	grams	cal.	grams	grams	grams	mg.	mg.	mg.	mg.	mg.	mg.	mg.
Spinach												
Raw, chopped	1 cup	55	15	2	Trace	2	51	259	0.06	0.11	0.3	28
Cooked from raw	1 cup	180	40	5	1	6	167	583	0.13	0.25	0.9	50
Cooked from frozen	1 cup	205	45	6	1	8	232	683	0.14	0.31	0.8	39
Squash												
Summer	1 cup	210	30	2	Trace	7	53	296	0.11	0.17	1.7	21
Winter	1 cup	205	130	4	1	32	57	945	0.10	0.27	1.4	27
Sweet potatoes	1 ea.	114	160	2	1	37	46	342	0.10	0.08	0.8	25
Tomatoes	1 ea.	135	25	1	Trace	6	16	300	0.07	0.05	0.9	28
Tomato catsup	1 tbsp.	15	15	Trace	Trace	4	3	54	0.01	0.01	0.2	2
Tomato juice, canned	1 glass	182	35	2	Trace	8	13	413	0.09	0.05	1.5	29
Turnips, cooked, diced	1 cup	155	35	1	Trace	8	54	291	0.06	0.08	0.5	34

Note: These figures represent the nutritive value of foods listed in the exact measurements, following traditional cooking methods. For more specific information, consult the product label. Dashes (—) denote lack of reliable data on measurable amounts.

RECOMMENDED DAILY ALLOWANCES

Sex/Age category	Age (yrs.)	Weight (lbs.)	Height (in.)	Food energy (calories)	Protein (grams)	Calcium (mg.)	Phosphorus (mg.)	Iron (mg.)	Vitamin A (Int. units)	Thiamin (mg.)	Riboflavin (mg.)	Niacin (mg.)	Ascorbic acid (mg.)
Infants	0–.5	14	24	lb. × 53.2	lb. × 1.0	360	240	10	1,400	0.3	0.4	5	35
	.5–1	20	28	lb. × 49.1	lb. × 0.9	540	400	15	2,000	0.5	0.6	8	35
Children	1–3	28	34	1,300	23	800	800	15	2,000	0.7	0.8	9	40
	4–6	44	44	1,800	30	800	800	10	2,500	0.9	1.1	12	40
	7–10	66	54	2,400	36	800	800	10	3,300	1.2	1.2	16	40
Males	11–14	97	63	2,800	44	1,200	1,200	18	5,000	1.4	1.5	18	45
	15–18	134	69	3,000	54	1,200	1,200	18	5,000	1.5	1.8	20	45
	19–22	147	69	3,000	54	800	800	10	5,000	1.5	1.8	20	45
	23–50	154	69	2,700	56	800	800	10	5,000	1.4	1.6	18	45
	51+	154	69	2,400	56	800	800	10	5,000	1.2	1.5	16	45
Females	11–14	97	62	2,400	44	1,200	1,200	18	4,000	1.2	1.3	16	45
	15–18	119	65	2,100	48	1,200	1,200	18	4,000	1.1	1.4	14	45
	19–22	128	65	2,100	46	800	800	18	4,000	1.1	1.4	14	45
	23–50	128	65	2,000	46	800	800	18	4,000	1.0	1.2	13	45
	51+	128	65	1,800	46	800	800	10	4,000	1.0	1.2	12	45
Pregnant				+300	+30	1,200	1,200	+18	5,000	+0.3	+0.3	+2	60
Lactating				+500	+20	1,200	1,200	18	6,000	+0.3	+0.5	+4	80

Source: Adapted from Recommended Dietary Allowances, 8th ed. (Washington: National Academy of Sciences–National Research Council, 1974).

Contributors

Dr. Enrico Arcelli is a European sports medicine authority. His chapter originally appeared in the West German magazine, *Leichtathletik*.

M. H. M. Arnold is a Britisher, who has done research at high altitudes in South America. His chapter originally appeared in the British magazine, *Athletics Weekly*.

George Beinhorn, former editor of *Bike World* magazine, has done research on yoga and diet.

Otto Brucker, M.D., is a Swiss authority on diet for athletes. His chapter was reprinted from the West German magazine, *Condition*.

Gary Chilton is a marathoner, who lives in Palo Alto, California.

Joe Henderson is a consulting editor to *Runner's World*, and is the author of many books, including *Jog, Run, Race*.

M. E. Houston was in the Department of Kinesiology at the University of Waterloo, in Ontario, Canada, at the time he wrote his chapter.

Ian Jackson, author of *Yoga and the Athlete,* is a former editor of *Soccer World* magazine.

Ludvig Prokop, M.D., is an Austrian sports medicine authority. His chapter originally appeared in the East German magazine, *Der Leichtathlet*.

George Sheehan, M.D., is a cardiologist, longtime medical editor for *Runner's World* magazine, and author of *Dr. Sheehan on Running*.

Stephen Streeter, who is a long-distance runner, is at Bates College in Lewiston, Maine. His chapter originally appeared in the March 1977 *Runner's World*.

Peter Van Handel works with Dr. David Costill in the Human Performance Laboratory at Ball State University. His chapter originally appeared in the July 1974 issue of *Runner's World*.

Index

Recommended Reading

Athletes Feet, editors of *Runner's World,* 1974.

Skin Care for the Athlete, Cameron Smith, 1978.

Basic Fitness Guide, Joe Owens, 1978.

Beginner's Running Guide, Hal Higdon, 1978.

Book for Every Body, Benny Crawford, 1978.

The Complete Diet Guide: For Runners and Other Athletes, Hal Higdon, ed., 1978.

The Complete Marathoner, Joe Henderson, ed., 1978.

The Complete Runner, editors of *Runner's World,* 1974.

The Complete Woman Runner, Richard Benyo, ed., 1978.

Encyclopedia of Athletic Medicine, George Sheehan, 1972.

New Exercises for Runners, editors of *Runner's World,* 1978.

The Female Runner, editors of *Runner's World,* 1974.

Food for Fitness, editors of *Bike World,* 1975.

The Foot Book: Advice for Athletes, Harry Hlavac, D.P.M., 1977.

Jog, Run, Race, Joe Henderson, 1977.

The Serious Runner's Handbook, Tom Osler, 1978.

Women's Running, Joan Ullyot, M.D., 1976.

Yoga and the Athlete, Ian Jackson, 1975.

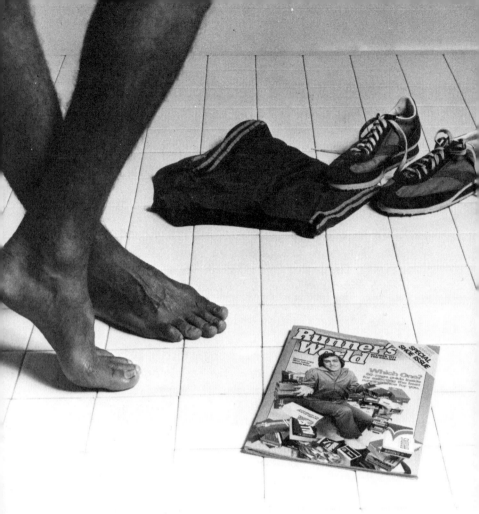

The runner's bare essentials*

Your shoes, your shorts, *Runner's World* and off you go into the world of running.

Runner's World **the nation's leading running publication,** has been covering the jogging/running scene since 1966. Articles for the beginning jogger through the competitive racer appear monthly. Every issue of ***Runner's World*** is loaded with good practical advice on medical problems, technical tips, equipment reviews, interviews with leading coaches & runners, and much more.

Come run with friends. Each month 510,000 fellow enthusiasts are sharing the information in the pages of ***Runner's World*** The joy of running is explored and expanded with each information packed issue—it's your coach and trainer making a monthly visit.

Exciting articles monthly: Fun Running, Run Better on Less Mileage, The Basics of Jogging, First Aid for the Injured, Running and Mental Health, Beginning Racing. Monthly columns by Dr. George Sheehan on medical advice, Dr. Joan Ullyot on women's running, Arthur Lydiard on training and racing.

Subscribe now for trouble-free miles of running. Just send $9.50 for 12 months or call (415) 965-3240 and charge to Master Charge or BankAmericard/Visa.

*Possibly because of climatic conditions or modesty you might want to add a shirt.

Runner's World Box 2680, Dept. 5534, Boulder, CO 80322